FIRST AID FOR THE® PSYCHIATRY CLERKSHIP

THIRD EDITION

LATHA GANTI STEAD, MD, MS, FACEP

Chief, Division of Clinical Research
Professor of Emergency Medicine
University of Florida College of Medicine at Gainesville
Gainesville, Florida
Adjunct Professor of Emergency Medicine
Mayo Clinic, College of Medicine
Rochester, Minnesota

MATTHEW S. KAUFMAN, MD

Assistant Professor of Medicine
Department of Hematology-Oncology
Albert Einstein College of Medicine
Bronx, New York
Resident, Emergency Medicine
Long Island Jewish Medical Center
New Hyde Park, New York

JASON YANOFSKI, MD

Forensic and Clinical Psychiatrist
Minor Traumatic Brain Injury (MTBI) Clinic
US Army Garrison
Bamberg, Germany
Psychiatry Residency
Johns Hopkins University Hospital
Baltimore, Maryland
Child Psychiatry Fellowship
University of Texas-Southwestern Medical Center
Dallas, Texas
Forensic Psychiatry Fellowship
Yale University
New Haven, Connecticut

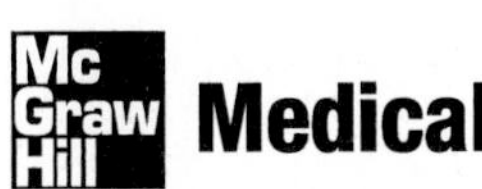

New York / Chicago / San Francisco / Lisbon / London / Madrid / Mexico City
Milan / New Delhi / San Juan / Seoul / Singapore / Sydney / Toronto

First Aid for the® Psychiatry Clerkship, Third Edition

1 2 3 4 5 6 7 8 9 0 QDB/QDB 14 13 12 11

ISBN 978-0-07-173923-8
MHID 0-07-173923-8

Notice

Medicine is an ever-changing science. As new research and clinical experience broaden our knowledge, changes in treatment and drug therapy are required. The authors and the publisher of this work have checked with sources believed to be reliable in their efforts to provide information that is complete and generally in accord with the standards accepted at the time of publication. However, in view of the possibility of human error or changes in medical sciences, neither the authors nor the publisher nor any other party who has been involved in the preparation or publication of this work warrants that the information contained herein is in every respect accurate or complete, and they disclaim all responsibility for any errors or omissions or for the results obtained from use of the information contained in this work. Readers are encouraged to confirm the information contained herein with other sources. For example and in particular, readers are advised to check the product information sheet included in the package of each drug they plan to administer to be certain that the information contained in this work is accurate and that changes have not been made in the recommended dose or in the contraindications for administration. This recommendation is of particular importance in connection with new or infrequently used drugs.

This book was set in Electra LH by Rainbow Graphics.
The editors were Catherine A. Johnson and Peter J. Boyle.
The production supervisor was Catherine Saggese.
Project management was provided by Tina Castle, Rainbow Graphics.
Quad/Graphics Dubuque was printer and binder.

This book is printed on acid-free paper.

Cataloging-in-publication data for this book is on file at the Library of Congress.

CONTENTS

ASSOCIATE EDITORS

S. SHANE KONRAD, MD
Clinical Assistant Professor
Department of Psychiatry
New York University School of Medicine
Division of Forensic Psychiatry
Bellevue Hospital Center
New York, New York

BRIAN COOKE, MD
Clinical Assistant Professor
Division of Forensic Psychiatry
Department of Psychiatry
University of Florida College of Medicine
Gainesville, Florida

CONTRIBUTING AUTHORS

NEIL KRISHAN AGGARWAL, MD, MBA, MA
Resident Physician, Department of Psychiatry
Yale University
New Haven, Connecticut
Anxiety and Adjustment Disorders

FRANK S. K. APPAH, JR., MD, PhD
Resident, Department of Psychiatry
Yale University School of Medicine
New Haven, Connecticut
Sleep Disorders

ALINA BOUZA, MD
Resident, Department of Psychiatry
Yale University School of Medicine
New Haven, Connecticut
Substance-Related Disorders

TRACY CABIBBO
Graduate Student in Microbiology
Fordham University
New York, New York
Mini Cases and Vignettes

NEDSON J. CAMPBELL, MD
Resident, Department of Psychiatry
Yale University School of Medicine
New Haven, Connecticut
Personality Disorders

BRIAN COOKE, MD
Clinical Assistant Professor
Division of Forensic Psychiatry
Department of Psychiatry
University of Florida College of Medicine
Gainesville, Florida
Forensic Psychiatry

GENEVIEVE A. HENRY, MD
Resident, Department of Psychiatry
Yale University School of Medicine
New Haven, Connecticut
Psychotic Disorders

CHRISTOPHER A. HOLLWEG, MPH
Class of 2011
St. George's University School of Medicine
Grenada
Mini Cases and Vignettes

PAVLE JOKSOVIC, MD
Resident, Department of Psychiatry
Yale University School of Medicine
New Haven, Connecticut
Somatoform and Factitious Disorders

S. SHANE KONRAD, MD
Clinical Assistant Professor
Department of Psychiatry
New York University School of Medicine
Division of Forensic Psychiatry
Bellevue Hospital Center
New York, New York
Forensic Psychiatry

KOURTNEY J. KOSLOSKY, MD
Resident, Yale University
Department of Psychiatry
New Haven, Connecticut
Impulse Control Disorders

MARI KURAHASHI, MD, MPH
Resident, Department of Psychiatry
Yale University
New Haven, Connecticut
Mood Disorders

CHRISTINA J. LEE, MD
Child Psychiatry Fellow
Yale University School of Medicine
Yale Child Study Center
New Haven, Connecticut
Psychiatric Disorders in Children

CARLA MARIENFELD, MD
Department of Psychiatry
Yale University
New Haven, Connecticut
Psychopharmacology

DAVID MATUSKEY, MD
Clinical Research Fellow
Neuroscience Research Training Program
Department of Psychiatry
Yale University
New Haven, Connecticut
Dissociative Disorders

MEREDITH ZOE NAIDORF, MD
Resident, Department of Psychiatry
Yale University
New Haven, Connecticut
Psychotherapies

MARK J. NICIU, JR., MD, PhD
Resident, Department of Psychiatry
Yale University
New Haven, Connecticut
Eating Disorders

SAMUEL O. SOSTRE, MD
Assistant Professor
Department of Psychiatry
Robert Wood Johnson Medical School
New Brunswick, New Jersey
Cognitive Disorders

AMELIA VILLAGOMEZ, MD
Resident, Department of Psychiatry
Yale University
New Haven, Connecticut
Examination and Diagnosis

PHILIP WILLIAMS, MD
Resident, Department of Psychiatry
Yale University
New Haven, Connecticut
Sexual Disorders

CYNTHIA N. WILSON, MD
Child and Adolescent Psychiatry Fellow
Yale University School of Medicine
New Haven, Connecticut
Psychiatric Disorders in Children

ERIN K. ZAHRADNIK, MD
Resident, Department of Psychiatry
Yale University
New Haven, Connecticut
Geriatric Psychiatry

FACULTY REVIEWERS

MADELON BARANOSKI, PhD
Associate Professor
Law and Psychiatry
Vice Chair HIC Committees II, IV
Human Research Protection Program
Yale University
New Haven, Connecticut

PATRICK K. FOX, MD
Assistant Professor of Psychiatry
Yale University School of Medicine
New Haven, Connecticut
Director, Whiting Forensic Division
Connecticut Valley Hospital
Middletown, Connecticut

DEBORAH KNUDSON GONZALEZ, MD
Assistant Professor
Department of Psychiatry
Yale University School of Medicine
New Haven, Connecticut

FREDERICK C. NUCIFORA, JR., PhD, DO, MHS
Assistant Professor
Department of Psychiatry
Johns Hopkins University School of Medicine
Baltimore, Maryland

KEVIN V. TRUEBLOOD, MD
Assistant Clinical Professor
Department of Psychiatry
Yale University School of Medicine
New Haven, Connecticut

PATRICIA ROY, MD
Department of Psychiatry
Johns Hopkins University School of Medicine
Baltimore, Maryland

Special thanks to
Dr. Thomas Brouette, MD, Psychiatry Clinical Clerkship Director, SUNY Downstate Medical Center, Brooklyn, New York

INTRODUCTION

This clinical study aid was designed in the tradition of the First Aid series of books. It is formatted in the same way as the other books in this series; however, a stronger clinical emphasis was placed on its content in relation to psychiatry. You will find that rather than simply preparing you for success on the clerkship exam, this resource will help guide you in the clinical diagnosis and treatment of many problems seen by psychiatrists.

Each of the chapters in this book contains the major topics central to the practice of psychiatry and has been specifically designed for the medical student learning level. It contains information that psychiatry clerks are expected to learn and will ultimately be responsible for on their shelf exams.

The content of the text is organized in the format similar to other texts in the First Aid series. Topics are listed by bold headings, and the "meat" of the topics provides essential information. The outside margins contain mnemonics, diagrams, exam and ward tips, summary or warning statements, and other memory aids. Exam tips are marked by the icon, tips for the wards by the icon, and clinical scenarios by the icon.

SECTION 1

How to Succeed in the Psychiatry Clerkship

The psychiatry clerkship can be very interesting and exciting.

A key to doing well in this clerkship is finding the balance between drawing a firm boundary of professionalism with your patients and creating a relationship of trust and comfort.

WHY SPEND TIME ON PSYCHIATRY?

For most of you reading this book, your medical school psychiatry clerkship will encompass the entirety of your formal training in psychiatry during your career in medicine.

Your awareness of the characteristics of mental dysfunction in psychiatric patients will serve you well in recognizing psychiatric symptoms in your patients no matter what field you specialize in.

Anxiety and depression can contribute to patients' medical conditions, and medical illnesses can cause significant psychological stress, revealing a previously subclinical psychiatric condition. The stress of extended hospitalizations alone can stress normal cognitive function beyond its adaptive reserve, resulting in transient psychiatric symptoms.

Psychotropic medications are common in the general population. Many of these drugs have significant potential medical side effects and drug interactions. You will become familiar with these during your clerkship and will encounter them in practice regardless of your field of medicine.

Because of the focus on spending time getting to know your patients, the psychiatry clerkship is an excellent time to practice your "bedside manner."

HOW TO BEHAVE ON THE WARDS

Respect the Patients

Always maintain professionalism and show the patients respect. Be respectful when discussing cases with your residents and attendings.

Respect the Field of Psychiatry

- Even if you aren't interested in psychiatry, do your best to show that you take the rotation seriously. Be aware of patients who try to split you from your team.
- You may not agree with all the decisions that your residents and attendings make, but it is important for everyone to be on the same page.
- Dress in a professional, conservative manner.
- Working with psychiatric patients can often be emotionally taxing. Keep yourself healthy.
- Psychiatry is a multidisciplinary field. It would behoove you to communicate with nurses, social workers and psychologists.
- Address patients formally unless otherwise told.

Take Responsibility for Your Patients

Know everything there is to know about your patients: their history, test results, details about their psychiatric and medical problems, and prognosis. Keep your intern or resident informed of new developments that they might not be aware of, and ask them for any updates you might not be aware of. Assist the team in developing a plan; speak to consultants and family. Never deliver bad news to patients or family members without the assistance of your supervising resident or attending.

Respect Patients' Rights

1. All patients have the right to have their personal medical information kept private. This means do not discuss the patient's information with family members without that patient's consent, and do not discuss any patient in hallways, elevators, or cafeterias.
2. All patients have the right to refuse treatment. This means they can refuse treatment by a specific individual (you, the medical student) or of a specific type (no electroconvulsive therapy). Patients can even refuse lifesaving treatment. The only exceptions to this rule are if the patient is deemed to not have the capacity to make decisions or understand situations, in which case a health care proxy should be sought, or if the patient is suicidal or homicidal.
3. All patients should be informed of the right to seek advance directives on admission. Often, this is done by the admissions staff, in a booklet. If your patient is chronically ill or has a life-threatening illness, address the subject of advance directives with the assistance of your attending.

Volunteer

Be self-propelled, self-motivated. Volunteer to help with a procedure or a difficult task. Volunteer to give a 20-minute talk on a topic of your choice. Volunteer to take additional patients. Volunteer to stay late.

Be a Team Player

Help other medical students with their tasks; teach them information you have learned. Support your supervising intern or resident whenever possible. Never steal the spotlight or make a fellow medical student look bad.

Keep Patient Information Handy

Use a clipboard, notebook, or index cards to keep patient information, including a miniature history and physical, and lab and test results, at hand.

Present Patient Information in an Organized Manner

Here is a template for the "bullet" presentation:

> "This is a [age]-year-old [gender] with a history of [major history such as bipolar disorder] who presented on [date] with [major symptoms, such as auditory hallucinations] and was found to have [working diagnosis]. [Tests

done] showed [results]. Yesterday, the patient [state important changes, new plan, new tests, new medications]. This morning the patient feels [state the patient's words], and the psychiatric and physical exams are significant for [state major findings]. Plan is [state plan].

The newly admitted patient generally deserves a longer presentation following the complete history and physical format.

Some patients have extensive histories. The whole history should be present in the admission note, but in ward presentation, it is often too much to absorb. In these cases, it will be very much appreciated by your team if you can generate a **good summary** that maintains an accurate picture of the patient. This usually takes some thought, but it's worth it.

HOW TO PREPARE FOR THE CLERKSHIP (SHELF) EXAM

If you have read about your core psychiatric illnesses and core symptoms, you will know a great deal about psychiatry. To study for the clerkship or shelf exam, we recommend:

2 or 3 weeks before exam: Read this entire review book, taking notes.
10 days before exam: Read the notes you took during the rotation on your core content list and the corresponding review book sections.
5 days before exam: Read this entire review book, concentrating on lists and mnemonics.
2 days before exam: Exercise, eat well, skim the book, and go to bed early.
1 day before exam: Exercise, eat well, review your notes and the mnemonics, and go to bed on time. Do not have any caffeine after 2 P.M.

Other helpful studying strategies include:

Study with Friends

Group studying can be very helpful. Other people may point out areas that you have not studied enough and may help you focus on the goal. If you tend to get distracted by other people in the room, limit this to less than half of your study time.

Study in a Bright Room

Find the room in your house or in your library that has the best, brightest light. This will help prevent you from falling asleep. If you don't have a bright light, get a halogen desk lamp or a light that simulates sunlight (not a tanning lamp).

Eat Light, Balanced Meals

Make sure your meals are balanced, with lean protein, fruits and vegetables, and fiber. A high-sugar, high-carbohydrate meal will give you an initial burst of energy for 1–2 hours, but then you'll drop.

Take Practice Exams

The point of practice exams is not so much the content that is contained in the questions, but the training of sitting still for 3 hours and trying to pick the best answer for each and every question.

Pocket Cards

The "cards" on the following page contain information that is often helpful in psychiatry practice. We advise that you make a photocopy of these cards, cut them out, and carry them in your coat pocket.

Mental Status Exam

Appearance: apparent age, attitude and behavior, eye contact, posture, dress and hygiene, psychomotor status
Speech: rate, volume, articulation
Emotions:
- *Mood:* patient's subjective emotional state—depressed, euphoric, anxious, sad, etc.
- *Affect:* objective emotional expression—expansive, labile, normal, constricted, blunted, flat, etc.

Thought:
- *Form:* organization of thoughts—circumstantial, tangential, linear, flight of ideas
- *Content:* content of thoughts—suicidal/homicidal ideation, delusions, preoccupations, hyperreligiosity

Perception: hallucinations, illusions, derealization, depersonalization
Cognition:
- *Level of consciousness:* alert, sleepy, lethargic
- *Orientation:* person, place, time
- *Attention/concentration:* serial 7s, spell "world" backwards
- *Memory:*
  - Registration: immediate recall of three objects
  - Short term: recall of objects after 5 minutes
  - Long term: ask about verifiable personal information
- *Fund of knowledge:* current events
- *Abstract thought:* interpretation of proverbs, analogies

Judgment: patient's ability to approach his/her problems in an appropriate manner
Insight: patient's awareness of his/her illness and need for treatment

Delirium

Characteristics: acute onset, waxing/waning sensorium (worse at night), disorientation, inattention, impaired cognition, disorganized thinking, delusions, altered sleep-wake cycle, perceptual disorder (hallucination, illusion)
Etiology: drugs (narcotics, benzodiazepines, anticholinergics, TCAs, steroids, Benadryl, etc.), EtOH withdrawal, metabolic (cardiac, respiratory, renal, hepatic, endocrine), infection, neurological causes (increased ICP, encephalitis, postictal, stroke)
Investigations:
- *Routine:* CBC, lytes, glucose, renal panel, UA, CXR, O_2 sat
- *Medium-yield:* ABG, LFTs, ECG (silent MI), ionized Ca^{2+}
- *If above inconclusive:* TFTs, Head CT/MRI, EEG, LP

Management: identify/correct underlying cause, simplify Rx regimen, d/c potentially offensive meds if possible, judiciously use neuroleptics, avoid benzodiazepines (except in EtOH withdrawal), create safe environment, provide reassurance/education, antipsychotics for acute agitation

Mini-Mental State Examination (MMSE)

Orientation (10):
- What is the [year] [season] [date] [day] [month]? (1 pt. each)
- Where are we [state] [county] [town] [hospital] [floor]?

Registration (3): Ask the patient to repeat three unrelated objects (1 pt. each on first attempt). If incomplete on first attempt, repeat up to six times (record # of trials).
Attention (5): Either serial 7s or "World" backwards (1 pt. for each correct letter or number).
Delayed recall (3): Ask patient to recall the three objects previously named (1 pt. each).
Language (9):
- Name two common objects, e.g., watch, pen (1 pt. each).
- Repeat the following sentence: "No ifs, ands, or buts" (1 pt.).
- Give patient blank paper. "Take it in your right hand, use both hands to fold it in half, and then put it on the floor" (1 pt. for each part correctly executed).
- Have patient read and follow: "Close your eyes" (1 pt.).
- Ask patient to write a sentence. The sentence must contain a subject and a verb, correct grammar and punctuation are not necessary (1 pt.)
- Ask the patient to copy the design. Each figure must have five sides, and two of the angles must intersect (1 pt.).

Mania ("DIG FAST")

Distractibility
Irritable mood/insomnia
Grandiosity
Flight of ideas
Agitation/increase in goal-directed activity
Speedy thoughts/speech
Thoughtlessness: seek pleasure without regard to consequences

Suicide Risk ("SAD PERSONS")

Sex—male
Age > 60 yrs
Depression
Previous attempt
Ethanol/drug abuse
Rational thinking loss
Suicide in family
Organized plan/access
No support
Sickness

Depression ("SIG E. CAPS")

Sleep
Interest
Guilt
Energy
Concentration
Appetite
Psychomotor Δs
Suicidal ideation
- Hopelessness
- Helplessness
- Worthlessness

First Aid for the® Psychiatry Clerkship, 3e; copyright © 2011 McGraw-Hill. All rights reserved.

Drugs of Abuse

Drug	Intoxication	Withdrawal
Alcohol Benzodiazepines	Disinhibition, mood lability, incoordination, slurred speech, ataxia, blackouts (EtOH), respiratory depression	Tremulousness, hypertension, tachycardia, anxiety, psychomotor agitation, nausea, seizures, hallucinations, DT (EtOH)
Barbiturates	Respiratory depression	Anxiety, seizures, delirium, life-threatening cardiovascular collapse
Opioids	CNS depression, nausea, vomiting, sedation, decreased pain perception, decreased GI motility, pupil constriction, respiratory depression	Increased sympathetic activity, N/V, diarrhea, diaphoresis, rhinorhea, piloerection, yawning, stomach cramps, myalgias, arthralgias, restlessness, anxiety, anorexia
Amphetamines Cocaine	Euphoria, increased attention span, aggressiveness, psychomotor agitation, pupil dilatation, hypertension, tachycardia, cardiac arrhythmias, psychosis (paranoia with amphetamines—formication with cocaine)	Post-use "crash": restlessness, headache, hunger, severe depression, insomnia/hypersomnia, strong psychological craving
PCP	Belligerence, impulsiveness, psychomotor agitation, vertical/horizontal nystagmus, hyperthermia, tachycardia, ataxia, psychosis, homicidality	May have recurrence of symptoms due to reabsorption in GI tract
LSD	Altered perceptual states (hallucinations, distortions of time and space), elevation of mood, "bad trips" (panic reaction), flashbacks (reexperience of the sensations in absence of drug use)	
Cannabis	Euphoria, anxiety, paranoia, slowed time, social withdrawal, increased appetite, dry mouth, amotivational syndrome	
Nicotine/ Caffeine	Restlessness, insomnia, anxiety, anorexia	Irritability, lethargy, headache, increased appetite, weight gain

Psychiatric Emergencies

Delirium Tremens (DTs):
- Typically within 2–4 days after cessation of EtOH but may occur later.
- Delirium, agitation, fever, autonomic hyperactivity, auditory and visual hallucinations.
- Treat aggressively with benzodiazepines and hydration.

Neuroleptic Malignant Syndrome (NMS):
- Fever, rigidity, autonomic instability, clouding of consciousness
- Withhold neuroleptics, hydrate, consider dantrolene
- Idiosyncratic, time-limited reaction

Serotonin Syndrome:
- Precipitated by use of two drugs with serotonin-enhancing properties (eg, MAOI + SSRI).
- Altered mental status, fever, agitation, tremor, myoclonus, hyperreflexia, ataxia, incoordination, diaphoresis, shivering, diarrhea.
- Discontinue offending agents, consider cyproheptadine.

Tyramine Reaction/Hypertensive Crisis:
- Precipitated by ingestion of tyramine containing foods while on MAOIs.
- Hypertension, headache, neck stiffness, sweating, nausea, vomiting, visual problems. Most serious consequences are stroke and possibly death.
- Treat with phentolamine.

Acute Dystonia:
- Early, sudden onset of muscle spasm: eyes, tongue, jaw, neck; may lead to laryngospasm requiring intubation.
- Treat with benztropine (Cogentin) or diphenhydramine (Benadryl).

Lithium Toxicity:
- May occur at any Li level (usually > 1.5).
- Nausea, vomiting, slurred speech, ataxia, incoordination, myoclonus, hyperreflexia, seizures, delirium, coma, nephrogenic diabetes insipidus
- Discontinue Li, hydrate aggressively, consider hemodialysis

Tricyclic Antidepressant (TCA) Toxicity:
- Primarily anticholinergic effects; cardiac conduction disturbances, hypotension, respiratory depression, agitation, hallucinations.
- CNS stimulation, depression, seizures.
- Monitor ECG—give bicarbonate for dysrhythmias and seizures, activated charcoal, cathartics, supportive treatment.

NOTES

SECTION II

High-Yield Facts

HIGH-YIELD FACTS IN

Examination and Diagnosis

Interviewing

MAKING THE PATIENT COMFORTABLE

The initial interview is of utmost importance to the psychiatrist. With practice, you will develop your own style and learn how to adapt the interview to the individual patient. In general, start the interview by asking open-ended questions and carefully note how the patient responds, as this is critical information for the mental status exam. Consider preparing for the interview by writing down the subheadings of the exam (see Figure 1-1). Find a safe area to conduct the interview. Use closed-ended questions to obtain the remaining pertinent information. During the first interview, the psychiatrist must establish a meaningful rapport with the patient in order to get accurate and pertinent information. This requires that questions be asked in a quiet, comfortable setting so that the patient is at ease. The patient should feel that the psychiatrist is interested, nonjudgmental, and compassionate. In psychiatry, the history is the most important factor in making a diagnosis and treatment plan.

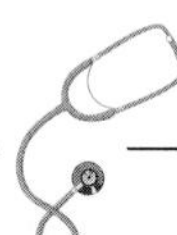

The HPI should include information about the current episode, including symptoms, duration, context, stressors, and impairment in function.

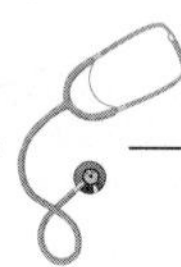

If you are seeing the patient in the ER, make sure to ask how they got to the ER (police, bus, walk-in, family member) and look to see what time they were triaged. For all initial evaluations, ask why the patient is seeking treatment *today* as opposed to any other day.

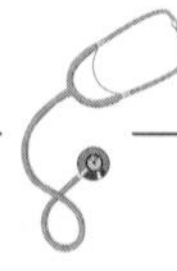

When taking a substance history, remember to ask about caffeine and nicotine use. If a heavy smoker is hospitalized and does not have access to nicotine replacement therapy, nicotine withdrawal may cause anxiety and agitation.

Taking the History

The psychiatric history follows a similar format as the history for other types of patients. It should include the following:

- Identifying data: The patient's name, sex, age, race, marital status, number of children, place and type of residence, occupation.
- Chief complaint (use the patient's own words). If called as a consultant, list reason for the consult.
- Sources of information.
- History of present illness (HPI):
  - *The 4 P's:* The patient's psychosocial and environmental conditions *predisposing to, precipitating, perpetuating,* and *protecting* against the current episode.
  - Information about previous episodes.
  - The patient's support system (whom the patient lives with, distance and level of contact with friends and relatives).
  - Vegetative symptoms (quality of sleep, appetite, psychomotor retardation/activation, concentration).
  - How work and relationship have been affected (for most diagnoses in the *Diagnostic and Statistical Manual of Mental Disorders,* 4th edition, Text Revision [DSM-IV-TR] there is a criterion that specifies that symptoms must cause clinically significant distress or impairment in social, occupational, or other important areas of functioning).
  - Relationship between physical and psychological symptoms.
  - Psychotic symptoms (eg, auditory and visual hallucinations).
  - Establish a baseline of mental health:
    - Patient's level of functioning when "well"
    - Life value, goals (outpatient setting)
- Past psychiatric history (include as applicable: history of suicide attempts, history of self harm (eg, cutting, burning oneself), psychiatric disorders in remission, medication trials, past psychiatric hospitalizations, current psychiatrist).

Date and Location:	
Identifying Patient Data:	
Chief Complaint:	Past Medical History:
History of Present Illness:	Allergies:
Past Psychiatric History:	Current Meds:
First contact:	Developmental History:
Diagnosis:	
Prior hospitalizations:	Relationships (children/marital status):
Suicide attempts:	
Outpatient treatment:	Education:
Med trials:	Work History:
Substance History:	Military History:
	Housing:
Smoking:	Income:
Family Psychiatric History:	Religion:
Legal History:	

FIGURE 1-1. Psychiatric History Outline.

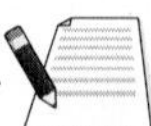

Importance of asking about OTC use: Nonsteroidal anti-inflammatories (NSAIDs) can ↓ lithium excretion → ↑ lithium concentrations (exceptions may be sulindac and aspirin).

- Substance history (participation in outpatient or inpatient drug rehab programs).
- Medical history (ask specifically about head trauma, seizures, pregnancy status).
- Family psychiatric and medical history (include treatment response as patient may respond similarly).
- Medications (ask about supplements and over-the-counter medications).
- Allergies: Clarify if it was a true allergy or an adverse drug event (eg, abdominal pain).
- Developmental history: Achieved developmental milestones on time, friends in school, performance academically.
- Social history: Include income source, employment, education, place of residence, who they live with, support system, religious affiliation and beliefs, legal history, amount of exercise, history of trauma or abuse).

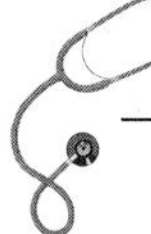

Psychomotor retardation, which refers to the slowness of voluntary and involuntary movements, may also be referred to as **hypokinesia** or **bradykinesia.** The term **akinesia** is used in extreme cases where absence of movement is observed.

Mrs. Gong is a 52-year-old Asian-American woman who arrives at the emergency room reporting that her deceased husband of 25 years told her that he would be waiting for her there. In order to meet him, she drove nonstop for 22 hours from a nearby state. She claims that her husband is a famous preacher and that she, too, has a mission from God. Although she does not specify the details of her mission, she says that she was given the ability to stop time until her mission is completed.

You evaluate Mrs. Gong and perform a mental status exam. Her **appearance** is that of a woman who looks older than her stated age. She is obese and unkempt. There is no evidence of tattoos or piercings. She has tousled hair and is dressed in a mismatched flowered skirt and a red T-shirt. Upon her arrival at the emergency room, her **behavior** is demanding, as she insists that you let her husband know that she has arrived. She then becomes irate and proceeds to yell, banging her head against the wall. She screams, "Stop hiding him from me!" She is uncooperative with redirection and is guarded during the remainder of the interview. Her **motor activity** is agitated.

She reports that her **mood** is "angry," and her **affect** as observed during the interview is labile and irritable. She reports experiencing high levels of energy despite not sleeping for 22 hours. She also reports that she has a history of psychiatric hospitalizations but refuses to provide further information.

Her **speech** is loud and pressured, with a foreign accent. Her **thought process** includes flight of ideas. Her **thought content** is significant for delusions of grandeur and thought broadcasting, as evidenced by her refusing to answer most questions claiming that you are able to know what she is thinking. She denies suicidal or homicidal ideation. She expresses **disturbances in perception** as she admits to frequent auditory hallucinations of command.

She is uncooperative with formal **cognitive function** testing, but you notice that she is oriented to place and person. However, she erroneously states that it is 1990. Her attention and concentration are notably impaired, as she appears distracted and frequently needs questions repeated. Her **insight** and **judgment** are determined to be poor.

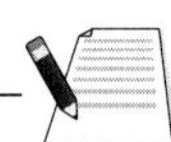

Automatisms are involuntary movements that occur during an altered state of consciousness and can range from purposeful to disorganized.

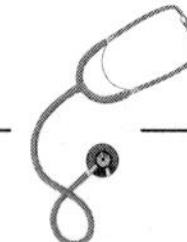

A hallmark of pressured speech is that it is usually uninterruptible and the patient is compelled to continue speaking.

You decide to admit Mrs. Gong to the inpatient psychiatric unit in order to allow for comprehensive diagnostic evaluation, the opportunity to obtain collateral information from her prior hospitalizations, safety monitoring, medical workup for possible reversible causes of her symptoms, and psychopharmacological treatment.

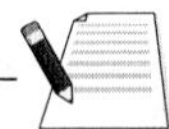

An example of inappropriate affect is a patient's laughing when being told he has a serious illness.

Mental Status Examination

This is analogous to performing a physical exam in other areas of medicine. It is the nuts and bolts of the psychiatric exam. It should describe the patient in as much detail as possible. The mental status exam assesses the following:

- Appearance/Behavior
- Speech
- Perception
- Sensorium/Cognition
- Insight/Judgment

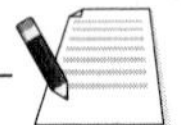

You can assess a patient's intellectual functioning by utilizing the *proverb interpretation* and *vocabulary* strategies. Proverb interpretation is helpful in assessing whether a patient has difficulty with abstraction. Being able to define a particular vocabulary word correctly and appropriately use it in a sentence should reflect a person's intellectual capacity.

The mental status exam tells only about the mental status at that moment; it can change every hour or every day, etc.

Appearance

- *Physical appearance:* Gender, age (looks older/younger than stated age), type of clothing, hygiene, posture, grooming, physical abnormalities, jewelry and cosmetic use, tattoos, level of consciousness (eg, alert, drowsy, lethargic, stuporous). Take specific notice of the following, which may be clues for possible diagnoses:
  - Pupil size: Drug intoxication/withdrawal.
  - Bruises in hidden areas: ↑ suspicion for abuse.
  - Needle marks/tracks: Drug use.
  - Eroding of tooth enamel: Eating disorders (from vomiting).
  - Superficial cuts on arms: Self-harm.
- *Behavior and psychomotor activity:* Mannerisms, tics, eye contact, activity level, psychomotor retardation/activation, akathisia, automatisms, catatonia, choreoathetoid movements, compulsions, dystonias, extrapyramidal symptoms, tardive dyskinesia, tremors.
- *Attitude:* Cooperative, seductive, flattering, charming, eager to please, entitled, controlling, uncooperative, hostile, guarded, critical, antagonistic, childish.

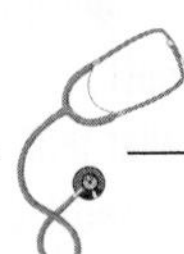

To assess mood, just ask, "How are you feeling today?" It is also helpful to have patients rate their stated mood on a scale of 1 to 10.

Speech

Rate (pressured, slowed, regular), rhythm (ie, prosody), articulation (stuttering), accent/dialect, modulation (loudness or softness), long or short latency of speech.

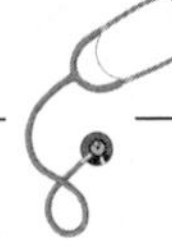

A patient who is laughing one second and crying the next has a *labile* affect.

Mood

Mood is the emotion that the patient tells you he feels or is conveyed nonverbally.

HIGH-YIELD FACTS

EXAMINATION AND DIAGNOSIS

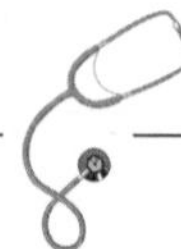

A patient who giggles while telling you that he set his house on fire and is facing criminal charges has an *inappropriate* affect.

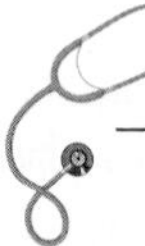

A patient who remains expressionless and monotone even when discussing extremely sad or happy moments in his life has a *flat* affect.

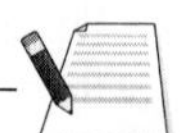

Examples of delusions:

- *Grandeur*—belief that one has special powers or is someone important (Jesus, president)
- *Paranoid*—belief that one is being persecuted
- *Reference*—belief that some event is uniquely related to patient (eg, a TV show character is sending patient messages)
- *Thought broadcasting*—belief that one's thoughts can be heard by others
- *Religious*—conventional beliefs exaggerated (eg, Jesus talks to me)
- *Somatic*—false belief concerning body image (eg, I cannot swallow)

AFFECT

Affect is an assessment of how the patient's mood appears to the examiner, including the amount and range of emotional expression. It is described with the following dimensions:

- *Quality* describes the depth and range of the feelings shown. Parameters: flat (none)—blunted (shallow)—constricted (limited)—full (average)—intense (more than normal).
- *Motility* describes how quickly a person appears to shift emotional states. Parameters: sluggish—supple—labile.
- *Appropriateness to content* describes whether the affect is congruent with the subject of conversation. Parameters: appropriate—not appropriate.

THOUGHT PROCESS

The patient's form of thinking—how he or she uses language and puts ideas together. It describes whether the patient's thoughts are logical, meaningful, and goal directed. It does not comment on *what* the patient thinks, only *how* the patient expresses his or her thoughts. Examples of disorders:

- **Loosening of associations:** No logical connection from one thought to another.
- **Flight of ideas:** Thoughts change abruptly from one idea to another, usually accompanied by rapid/pressured speech.
- **Neologisms:** Made-up words.
- **Word salad:** Incoherent collection of words.
- **Clang associations:** Word connections due to phonetics rather than actual meaning. "My car is red. I've been in bed. It hurts my head."
- **Thought blocking:** Abrupt cessation of communication before the idea is finished.
- **Tangentiality:** Point of conversation never reached due to lack of goal-directed associations between ideas; responses usually in the ballpark.
- **Circumstantiality:** Point of conversation is eventually reached but with overinclusion of trivial or irrelevant details.

THOUGHT CONTENT

Describes the types of ideas expressed by the patient. Examples of disorders:

- **Poverty of thought versus overabundance:** Too few versus too many ideas expressed.
- **Delusions:** Fixed, false beliefs that are not shared by the person's culture and cannot be changed by reasoning. Delusions are classified as bizarre (impossible to be true) or nonbizarre (at least possible).
- **Suicidal and homicidal thoughts:** Ask if the patient feels like harming him/herself or others. Identify if the plan is well formulated. Ask if the patient has an intent (ie, if released right now, would he go and kill himself or harm others?). Ask if the patient has means to kill himself (firearms in the house/multiple prescription bottles).
- **Phobias:** Persistent, irrational fears.
- **Obsessions:** Repetitive, intrusive thoughts.
- **Compulsions:** Repetitive behaviors (usually linked with obsessive thoughts).

PERCEPTION

- *Hallucinations*: Sensory perception that occur in the absence of an actual stimulus.
  - Describe the sensory modality: auditory (most common), visual, taste, olfactory, or tactile.
  - Describe the details (eg, auditory hallucinations may be ringing, humming, whispers, or voices speaking clear words). Command auditory hallucinations are voices that instruct the patient to do something.
  - Ask if the hallucination is experienced only before falling asleep (hypnagogic hallucination) or upon awakening (hypnopompic hallucination).
- *Illusions:* Inaccurate perception of existing sensory stimuli (eg, wall appears as if it's moving).

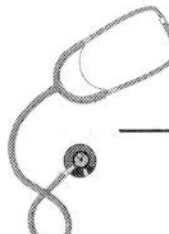

The following question can help screen for compulsions: Do you clean, check, or count things on a repetitive basis?

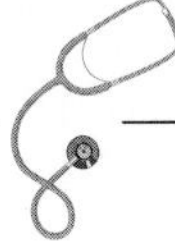

An auditory hallucination that instructs a patient to harm himself or others is an important risk factor for suicide or homicide.

SENSORIUM AND COGNITION

Sensorium and cognition are assessed in the following ways:

- **Consciousness:** Patient's level of awareness; possible range includes: Alert—drowsy—lethargic—stuporous—coma.
- **Orientation:** To person, place, and time.
- **Calculation:** Ability to add/subtract.
- **Memory:**
  - Immediate (registration)—dependent on attention/concentration and can be tested by asking a patient to repeat several digits or words.
  - Recent (short-term memory)—events within the past few hours or days.
  - Remote memory (long-term memory).
- **Fund of knowledge:** Level of knowledge in the context of the patient's culture and education (eg, Who is the president? Who was Picasso?).
- **Attention/Concentration:** Ability to subtract serial 7s from 100 or to spell "world" backwards.
- **Reading/Writing:** Simple sentences (must make sure the patient is literate first!).
- **Abstract concepts:** Ability to explain similarities between objects and understand the meaning of simple proverbs.

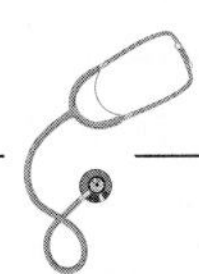

Alcoholic hallucinosis refers to hallucinations (usually visual, although auditory and tactile may occur) that develop within 12–24 hours of abstinence from alcohol (in an alcohol-dependent person) and resolve within 24–48 hours. Patients usually are aware that these hallucinations are not real. In contrast to delirium tremens (DTs), there is no clouding of sensorium and vital signs are normal.

INSIGHT

Insight is the patient's level of awareness and understanding of his or her problem. Problems with insight include complete denial of illness or blaming it on something else. Insight can be described as full, partial/limited, or none.

JUDGMENT

Judgment is the patient's ability to understand the outcome of his or her actions and use this awareness in decision making. In addition to information from the HPI (eg, how a patient was brought to treatment or medication compliance), you can ask hypothetical questions such as, "What would you do if you smelled smoke in a crowded movie theater?" Judgment can be described as excellent, good, fair, or poor.

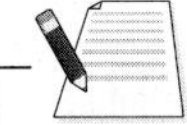

Think: hypno**POmP**ic occurs when you **POP** out of bed.

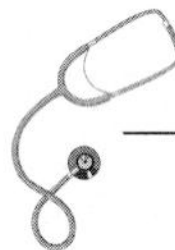

To test ability to abstract, ask:

1. Similarities: How are an apple and orange alike? (Normal answer: "They are fruits." *Concrete* answer: "They are round.")
2. Proverb testing: What is meant by the phrase, "You can't judge a book by it's cover?" (Normal answer: "You can't judge people just by how they look." *Concrete* answer: "Books have different covers.")

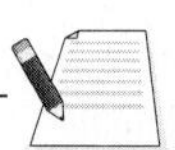

Keep it straight! DSM-IV is a multiaxial diagnosis system.

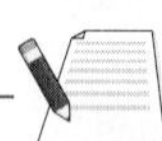

Axis I describes clinical disorders.
Axis II describes developmental and personality disorders.
Axis III describes physical disorders.
Axis IV describes the severity of psychosocial factors.
Axis V provides a global assessment.

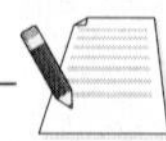

A prior history of violence is the most important predictor of future violence.

Mini-Mental State Examination (MMSE)

The MMSE is a simple, brief test used to assess gross cognitive functioning. See the Cognitive Disorders chapter for detailed description. The areas tested include:

- Orientation (to person, place, and time).
- Memory (immediate—registering three words; and recent—recalling three words 5 minutes later).
- Concentration and attention (serial 7s, spell "world" backwards).
- Language (naming, repetition, comprehension).
- Reading and writing.
- Visuospatial ability (copy of design).

INTERVIEWING SKILLS

General Approaches to Types of Patients

Violent Patient

One should avoid being alone with a potentially violent patient. Inform staff of your whereabouts. Know if there are accessible panic buttons. To assess violence or homicidality, one can simply ask, "Do you feel like you want to hurt someone or that you might hurt someone?" If the patient expresses imminent threats against friends, family, or others, the doctor should notify potential victims and/or protection agencies when appropriate (Tarasoff rule).

Delusional Patient

Although the psychiatrist should not directly challenge a delusion or insist that it is untrue, he should not imply he believes it either. He should simply acknowledge that he understands the *patient* believes the delusion is true.

Depressed Patient

A depressed patient may be skeptical that he or she can be helped. It is important to offer reassurance that he or she can improve with appropriate therapy. Inquiring about suicidal thoughts is crucial; a feeling of hopelessness, substance use, and/or a history of prior suicide attempts reveal an ↑ risk for suicide. If the patient is planning or contemplating suicide, he or she must be hospitalized or otherwise protected.

DIAGNOSIS AND CLASSIFICATION

Diagnosis as per DSM-IV-TR Multiaxial Classification Scheme

The American Psychiatric Association uses a multiaxial classification system for diagnoses. Criteria and codes for each diagnosis are outlined in their DSM-IV-TR.

Axis I: All diagnoses of mental illness (including substance abuse and developmental disorders), not including personality disorders and mental retardation.
Axis II: Personality disorders and mental retardation.
Axis III: General medical conditions.

TABLE 1-1. Global Assessment of Function (GAF) Scale

1–10	11–20	21–30	31–40	41–50	51–60	61–70	71–80	81–90	91–100
Persistent danger of severely hurting self or others. *Recurrent violence.*	Gross impairment in communication. *Largely incoherent or mute.*	Behavior is considerably influenced by delusions or hallucinations.	Some impairment in reality testing or communication. *Speech is at times illogical, obscure, or irrelevant.*	Serious symptoms. *Suicidal ideation, severe obsessional rituals, frequent shoplifting.*	Moderate symptoms. *Flat affect and circumstantial speech, occasional panic attacks.*	Some mild symptoms. *Depressed mood, mild insomnia.*	If symptoms are present, they are transient and expectable reactions to psychosocial stressors. *Difficulty concentrating after family argument.*	Absent or minimal symptoms. *Mild anxiety before an exam. Generally satisfied with life. No more than everyday problems or concerns. Occasional argument with family members.*	No symptoms.
Serious suicidal act with clear expectation of death.	Some danger of hurting self or others. *Suicide attempts without clear expectation of death, frequently violent, manic excitement.*	Serious impairment in communication or judgment. *Sometimes incoherent, acts grossly inappropriately, suicidal preoccupation.*	Major impairment in several areas, such as work or school, family relations, judgment, thinking, or mood. *Depressed man avoids friends, neglects family, and is unable to work. Child frequently beats up younger children, is defiant at home and is failing in school.*	Any serious impairment in social, occupational, or school functioning. *No friends, unable to keep a job.*	Moderate difficulty in social, occupational, or school functioning. *Few friends, conflicts with coworkers.*	Some difficulty in social, occupational, or school functioning. *Occasional truancy, or theft within the household, but generally functioning pretty well, has some meaningful interpersonal relationships.*	No more than slight impairment in social, occupational, or school functioning. *Temporarily falling behind in school work.*	Good functioning in all areas, interested and involved in a wide range of activities, socially effective.	Superior functioning in a wide range of activities. *Life's problems never seem to get out of hand.*
Persistent inability to maintain minimal personal hygiene.	Occasionally fails to maintain minimal personal hygiene. *Smears feces.*	Inability to function in almost all areas. *Stays in bed all day, no job, home, or friends.*							Sought out by others because of his or her many positive qualities.

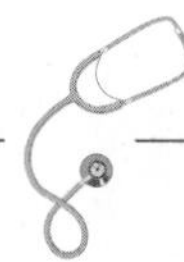

In assessing suicidality, do not simply ask, "Do you want to hurt yourself?" because this does not directly address suicidality (he may plan on dying in a painless way). Ask directly about killing self or suicide. If contemplating suicide, ask the patient if he has a plan of how to do it and if he has intent; a detailed plan, intent, and the means to accomplish it suggest a serious threat.

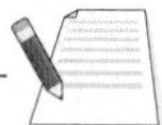

The Minnesota Multiphasic Personality Inventory (MMPI) is an objective psychological test that is used to assess a person's personality and identify psychopathologies. The mean score is 50 and the standard deviation is 10.

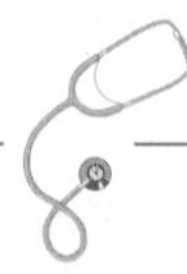

IQ Chart

Very superior: > 130
Superior: 120–129
High average: 110–119
Average: 90–109
Low average: 80–89
Borderline: 70–79
Mild mental retardation: 50–70
Moderate mental retardation: 35–49
Severe mental retardation: 25–34
Profound mental retardation: < 2

Axis IV: Psychosocial and environmental problems (eg, homelessness, divorce, etc.).
Axis V: The Global Assessment of Function (GAF), which rates overall level of daily functioning (social, occupational, and psychological) on a scale of 0 to 100. (See Table 1-1). Rate current GAF vs. high GAF during the past year. In general, a criterion for hospitalization is a GAF of ≤ 30.

DIAGNOSTIC TESTING

Intelligence Tests

Aspects of intelligence include memory, logical reasoning, ability to assimilate factual knowledge, understanding of abstract concepts, etc.

INTELLIGENCE QUOTIENT (IQ)

IQ is a test of intelligence with a mean of 100 and a standard deviation of 100. These scores are adjusted for age. An IQ of 100 signifies that mental age equals chronological age and corresponds to the 50th percentile in intellectual ability for the general population.

Intelligence tests assess cognitive function by evaluating comprehension, fund of knowledge, math skills, vocabulary, picture assembly, and other verbal and performance skills. Two common tests are:

Wechsler Adult Intelligence Scale (WAIS):
- Most common test for ages 16–75.
- Assesses overall intellectual functioning.
- Two parts: Verbal and visual-spatial.

Stanford-Binet Test: Tests intellectual ability in patients ages 2–18.

Objective Personality Assessment Tests

These tests are questions with standardized-answer format that can be objectively scored. The following is an example:

Minnesota Multiphasic Personality Inventory (MMPI-2)
- Tests personality for different pathologies and behavioral patterns.
- Most commonly used.

Projective (Personality) Assessment Tests

Projective tests have no structured-response format. The tests often ask for interpretation of ambiguous stimuli. Examples are:

Thematic Apperception Test (TAT)
- Test taker creates stories based on pictures of people in various situations.
- Used to evaluate motivations behind behaviors.

Rorschach Test
- Interpretation of inkblots.
- Used to identify thought disorders and defense mechanisms.

HIGH-YIELD FACTS IN

Psychotic Disorders

PSYCHOSIS

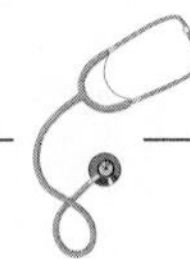

Psychosis is exemplified by either delusions, hallucinations, or severe disorganization of thought/behavior.

Psychosis is a general term used to describe a distorted perception of reality. Poor reality testing may be accompanied by delusions, perceptual disturbances (illusions or hallucinations), and/or disorganized thinking. Psychosis can be a symptom of schizophrenia, mania, and severe depression, and it can be substance induced. Hallucinations and delusions are also frequently observed in delirium and dementia.

DELUSIONS

Delusions are fixed, false beliefs that cannot be altered by rational arguments and cannot be accounted for by the cultural background of the individual.

They can be categorized as either bizarre or nonbizarre. A *nonbizarre* delusion is a belief that could be true but just isn't. Example: "The neighbors are reading my mail, and my wife is having an affair." A *bizarre* delusion is a false belief that is impossible. Example: "A Martian fathered my baby and inserted a microchip in my brain."

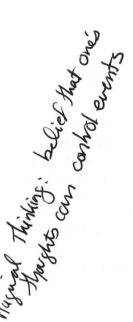

Delusions can also be categorized by theme:

- **Delusions of persecution/paranoid delusions:** Irrational belief that one is being persecuted. Example: "The CIA is after me and tapped my phone."
- **Ideas of reference:** Belief that cues in the external environment are uniquely related to the individual. Example: "Jesus is speaking to me through TV characters."
- **Delusions of control:** Includes **thought broadcasting** (belief that one's thoughts can be heard by others) and **thought insertion** (belief that other people thoughts are being placed in one's head).
- **Delusions of grandeur:** Belief that one has special powers beyond those of a normal person. Example: "I am the all-powerful son of God and I shall bring down my wrath on you if I don't get my way."
- **Delusions of guilt:** False belief that one is guilty or responsible for something. Example: "I am responsible for all the world's wars."
- **Somatic delusions:** False belief that one is infected with a disease or has a certain illness.

PERCEPTUAL DISTURBANCES

Auditory hallucinations that directly tell the patient to perform certain acts are called **command hallucinations.**

- **Illusion:** Misinterpretation of an existing sensory stimulus (such as mistaking a shadow for a cat).
- **Hallucination:** Sensory perception without an actual external stimulus.
  - **Auditory:** Most commonly exhibited by schizophrenic patients.
  - **Visual:** Less common in schizophrenia. May accompany drug intoxication, drug and alcohol withdrawal, or delirium.
  - **Olfactory:** Usually an aura associated with epilepsy.
  - **Tactile:** Usually secondary to drug abuse or alcohol withdrawal.

DIFFERENTIAL DIAGNOSIS OF PSYCHOSIS

- Psychosis secondary to general medical condition
- Substance-induced psychotic disorder
- Delirium/Dementia
- Bipolar disorder, manic/mixed episode
- Major depression with psychotic features
- Brief psychotic disorder
- Schizophrenia
- Schizophreniform disorder
- Schizoaffective disorder
- Delusional disorder

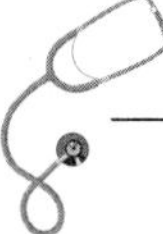

It's important to be able to distinguish between delusion, illusion, and hallucination. A **delusion** is a false belief; an **illusion** is misinterpretation of an external stimulus, and **hallucination** is perception in the absence of an external stimulus.

PSYCHOSIS SECONDARY TO GENERAL MEDICAL CONDITION

Medical causes of psychosis include:

1. *Central nervous system (CNS) disease* (cerebrovascular disease, multiple sclerosis, neoplasm, Alzheimer disease, Parkinson disease, Huntington chorea, tertiary syphilis, temporal lobe epilepsy, encephalitis, prion disease, neurosarcoidosis, AIDS).
2. *Endocrinopathies* (Addison/Cushing disease, hyper/hypothyroidism, hyper/hypocalcemia, hypopituitarism).
3. *Nutritional/Vitamin deficiency states* (B_{12}, folate, niacin).
4. *Other* (connective tissue disease [systemic lupus erythematosus, temporal arteritis], porphyria).

DSM-IV criteria for psychotic disorder secondary to a general medical condition include:

- Prominent hallucinations or delusions.
- Symptoms do not occur only during episode of delirium.
- Evidence to support medical cause from lab data, history, or physical.

Elderly, medically ill patients who present with psychotic symptoms such as hallucinations, confusion, or paranoia should be carefully evaluated for delirium, which is a far more common finding in this population.

PSYCHOSIS SECONDARY TO MEDICATION OR SUBSTANCE USE

Prescription medications that may cause psychosis in some patients include corticosteroids, antiparkinsonian agents, anticonvulsants, antihistamines, anticholingerics, some antihypertensives including beta blockers, digitalis, methylphenidate, and flouroquinolones. Other substances such as alcohol, cocaine, hallucinogens (LSD, Ecstasy), marijuana, benzodiazepines, barbiturates, and phencyclidine (PCP) are also known to cause psychosis.

DSM-IV CRITERIA

- Prominent hallucinations or delusions.
- Symptoms do not occur only during episode of delirium.
- Evidence to support medication or substance-related cause from lab data, history, or physical.
- Disturbance is not better accounted for by a psychotic disorder that is not substance induced.

Derealization: subjective sense that environment is strange or unreal

Depersonalization: feeling that one is not one's self

SCHIZOPHRENIA

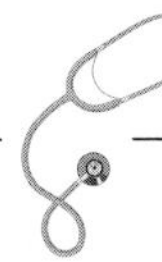

To make the diagnosis of schizophrenia, a patient must have symptoms of the disease for at least 6 months.

A 24-year-old male graduate student without prior medical or psychiatric history is reported by his mother to have been very anxious over the past 6 months, with increasing concern that people are watching him. He now claims to "hear voices" telling him what must be done to "fix the country." *Important workup?* Thyroid-stimulating hormone (TSH), rapid plasma reagin (RPR), brain imaging. *Likely diagnosis?* Paranoid schizophrenia. *Next step?* Antipsychotics.

Schizophrenia is a psychiatric disorder characterized by a constellation of abnormalities in thinking, emotion, and behavior. There is no single symptom that is pathognomonic, and there is a diverse clinical presentation. Schizophrenia is usually chronic, with significant psychosocial and medical consequences to the patient.

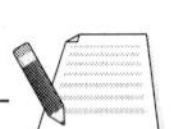

Think of positive symptoms as things that are **ADDED** onto normal behavior. Think of negative symptoms as things that are **SUBTRACTED** or missing from normal behavior.

Positive, Negative, and Cognitive Symptoms

In general, the symptoms of schizophrenia are broken up into three categories:

- **Positive symptoms:** Hallucinations, delusions, bizarre behavior, disorganized speech. These tend to respond more robustly to the current antipsychotic medications.
- **Negative symptoms:** Blunted affect, anhedonia, apathy, alogia, and lack of interest in socialization. These symptoms are often treatment resistant and contribute significantly to the social isolation of schizophrenic patients.
- **Cognitive symptoms:** Impairments in attention, executive function, and working memory. These symptoms may → poor work and school performance.

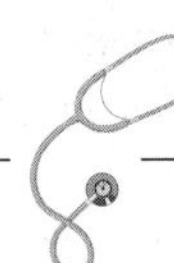

Stereotyped movement, bizarre posturing, and muscle rigidity are seen in catatonic schizophrenic patients.

Three Phases

Symptoms of schizophrenia usually present in three phases:

1. **Prodromal:** Decline in functioning that precedes the first psychotic episode. The patient may become socially withdrawn and irritable. He or she may have physical complaints and/or newfound interest in religion or the occult.
2. **Psychotic:** Perceptual disturbances, delusions, and disordered thought process/content.
3. **Residual:** Occurs between episodes of psychosis. It is marked by flat affect, social withdrawal, and odd thinking or behavior (negative symptoms). Patients can continue to have hallucinations even with treatment.

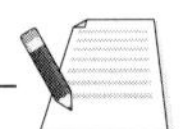

Clozapine is typically considered when a patient fails both typical and atypical antipsychotics.

Diagnosis of Schizophrenia

DSM-IV Criteria

- *Two or more* of the following must be present for at least *1 month:*
  1. Delusions
  2. Hallucinations
  3. Disorganized speech
  4. Grossly disorganized or catatonic behavior
  5. Negative symptoms (such as flattened affect)

  Note: Only *one* of the above symptoms are required if delusions are bizarre or hallucinations consist of a voice keeping up a running commentary on the person's behavior or thoughts, or two or more voices conversing with each other.
- Must cause significant social or occupational functional deterioration.
- Duration of illness for at least 6 months (including prodromal or residual periods in which above criteria may not be met).
- Symptoms not due to medical, neurological, or substance-induced disorder.

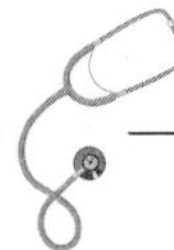

The 5 **A**'s of schizophrenia (negative symptoms):
1. **A**nhedonia
2. **A**ffect (flat)
3. **A**logia (poverty of speech)
4. **A**volition (apathy)
5. **A**ttention (poor)

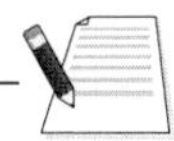

Types of Schizophrenia

Paranoid type: Characterized by delusions and auditory hallucinations.

Disorganized type: Characterized by disorganized speech, behavior and flat or inappropriate affect.

Catatonic type: Characterized by rigid posture, inappropriate or repetitive and purposeless movements, echolalia (repeating what someone else says), and echopraxia (copying what someone else does).

Residual type: Prominent negative symptoms.

Undifferentiated type: Doesn't fulfill any of the other criteria.

Subtypes of Schizophrenia

Patients are further subdivided into the following five subtypes:

1. **Paranoid type:** Often higher functioning, older age of onset. Must meet the following criteria:
   - Preoccupation with one or more delusions or frequent auditory hallucinations.
   - No predominance of disorganized speech, disorganized or catatonic behavior, or inappropriate affect.
2. **Disorganized type:** Poor functioning type, early onset. Must meet the following criteria:
   - Disorganized speech
   - Disorganized behavior
   - Flat or inappropriate affect
3. **Catatonic type:** Rare. Must meet at least two of the following criteria:
   - Motor immobility
   - Excessive purposeless motor activity
   - Extreme negativism or mutism
   - Peculiar voluntary movements or posturing
   - **Echolalia** or **echopraxia**
4. **Undifferentiated type:** Characteristic of more than one subtype or none of the subtypes.
5. **Residual type:** Prominent *negative* symptoms (such as flattened affect or social withdrawal) with only minimal evidence of positive symptoms (such as hallucinations or delusions).

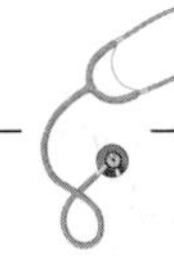

Echolalia—repeats words or phrases

EchoPRAxia—mimics behavior (**PRA**ctices behavior)

Mr. Torres is a 21-year-old man who is brought to the ER by his mother after he began talking about "aliens" who were trying to steal his soul. Mr. Torres reports that "aliens" left messages for him by arranging sticks outside his home and sometimes sent thoughts into his mind. On exam, he is guarded and often stops talking while in the middle of expressing a thought. Mr. Torres

(continued)

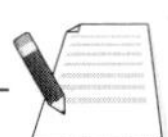

Brief psychotic disorder lasts for < 1 month. Schizophreniform disorder can last between 1 and 6 months. Schizophrenia lasts > 6 months.

appears anxious and frequently scans the room for "aliens," which he thinks may have followed him to the hospital. He denies any plan to harm himself, but admits that the "aliens" sometimes want him to throw himself in front of a car, "as this will change the systems that belong under us."

The patient's mother reports that he began expressing these ideas a few months ago, but that they have become more severe in the last few weeks. She reports that during the past year, he has become isolated from his peers, frequently talks to himself, and has stopped going to community college. He has also spent most of his time reading science fiction books and creating devices that will prevent "aliens" from hurting him. She reports that she is concerned because the patient's father, who left while the patient was a child, exhibited similar symptoms many years ago and has spent most of his life in psychiatric hospitals.

What is Mr. Torres's most likely diagnosis? What differential diagnoses should be considered?

Mr. Torres's most likely diagnosis is schizophrenia, paranoid type. He exhibits delusional ideas that are bizarre and paranoid in nature. He also reports the presence of frequent auditory hallucinations and disturbances in thought process, that included thought blocking. Although the patient's mother reported that his psychotic symptoms began "a few months ago," the patient had exhibited social and occupational dysfunction during the last year. Mr. Torres quit school, became isolated and had been responding to internal stimuli since that time. In addition, his father appears to also suffer from a psychotic disorder. In this case, it appears that the disorder has been present for more than 6 months; however, if this is unclear, the diagnosis of schizophreniform disorder is instead made.

The differential diagnosis should also include schizoaffective disorder, substance-induced psychotic disorder, psychosis due to medical condition, mood disorder with psychotic features, and delusional disorder.

What would be appropriate steps in the acute management of this patient?

Treatment would include inpatient hospitalization in order to provide a safe environment with monitoring of suicidal ideation secondary to his psychosis. Routine laboratory tests, including a urine or serum drug screening, should be undertaken. The patient should begin treatment with antipsychotic medication while closely monitoring for potential side effects.

Psychiatric Exam of Schizophrenics

The typical findings in schizophrenic patients on exam include:

- Disheveled appearance
- Flattened affect
- Disorganized thought process
- Intact memory and orientation
- Auditory hallucinations
- Paranoid delusions
- Ideas of reference (feel references are being made to them by the television or newspaper, etc)
- Concrete understanding of similarities/proverbs
- Lack insight into their disease

Epidemiology

- Schizophrenia affects approximately 1% of people over their lifetime.
- Men and women are equally affected but have different presentations and outcomes:
  - Men tend to present around 20 years of age.
  - Women present closer to 30 years of age.
- Men tend to have more negative symptoms and more impaired social functioning compared to women.
- Schizophrenia rarely presents before age 15 or after age 55.
- There is a strong genetic predisposition:
  - 50% concordance rate among monozygotic twins
  - 40% risk of inheritance if both parents have schizophrenia
  - 12% risk if one first-degree relative is affected
- Substance abuse is comorbid with schizophrenia in many patients. The most commonly abused substance is alcohol (30–50%), followed by cannabis (15–20%) and cocaine (5–10%).
- Postpsychotic depression is the phenomenon of schizophrenic patients developing a major depressive episode after resolution of their psychotic symptoms.

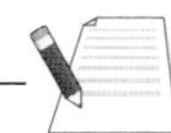

People born in winter and early spring have a higher incidence of schizophrenia for unknown reasons. (One theory involves seasonal variation in viral infections, particularly second trimester exposure to influenza virus.)

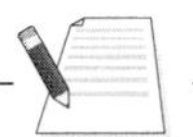

Schizophrenia is found in lower socioeconomic groups due to "downward drift" (they have difficulty in holding good jobs, so they tend to drift downward socioeconomically).

Downward Drift

Lower socioeconomic groups have higher rates of schizophrenia. This may be due to the **downward drift hypothesis,** which postulates that people suffering from schizophrenia are unable to function well in society and hence enter lower socioeconomic groups. Many homeless people in urban areas suffer from schizophrenia.

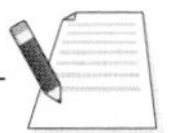

Akathisia is an unpleasant, subjective sense of restlessness often manifested by the inability to sit still.

Pathophysiology of Schizophrenia: The Dopamine Hypothesis

Though the exact cause of schizophrenia is not known, it appears to be partly related to ↑ dopamine activity in certain neuronal tracts. Evidence to support this hypothesis is that most antipsychotics that are successful in treating schizophrenia are dopamine receptor antagonists. In addition, cocaine and amphetamines ↑ dopamine activity and can → schizophrenic-like symptoms.

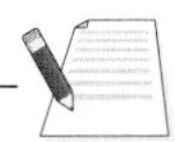

The lifetime prevalence of schizophrenia is around 1%.

Theorized Dopamine Pathways Affected in Schizophrenia

- *Prefrontal cortical:* Inadequate dopaminergic activity responsible for negative symptoms.
- *Mesolimbic:* Excessive dopaminergic activity responsible for positive symptoms.

Other Important Dopamine Pathways Affected by Neuroleptics

- *Tuberoinfundibular:* Blocked by neuroleptics, causing hyperprolactinemia, which may → gynecomastia, galactorrhea, and menstrual irregularities.
- *Nigrostriatal:* Blocked by neuroleptics, causing extrapyramidal side effects such as tremor, slurred speech, akathisia, dystonia, and other abnormal movements.

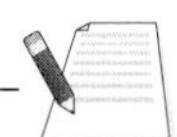

Schizophrenia has a very large genetic component. If one identical twin has schizophrenia, the risk of the other identical twin having schizophrenia is 50%. Moreover, a biological child of schizophrenic person has a higher chance of schizophrenia, even if he is adopted.

Schizophrenics have enlarged ventricles and prominent sulci

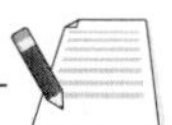

Computed tomographic (CT) scans of patients with schizophrenia may show enlargement of the ventricles and diffuse cortical atrophy.

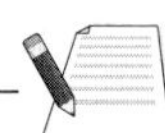

Significant improvement is noted in 70% of schizophrenic patients who take antipsychotic medication.

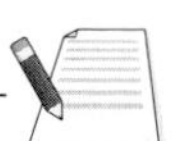

Deafness is a predisposing factor to paranoid psychosis.

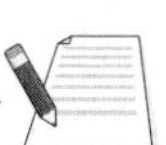

Schizophrenia often involves neologisms. **Neologism** is use of words that have meaning only to the person who uses them and is different than the orthodox meaning of the word.

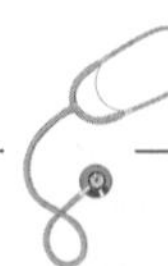

First-generation antipsychotic medications are also referred to as typical or conventional neuroleptics. Second-generation antipsychotic medications are referred to as atypical neuroleptics.

Other Neurotransmiter Abnormalities Implicated in Schizophrenia

- **Elevated serotonin:** Some of the atypical antipsychotics (such as risperidone and clozapine) antagonize serotonin and weakly antagonize dopamine.
- **Elevated norepinephrine:** Long-term use of antipsychotics has been shown to ↓ activity of noradrenergic neurons.
- **↓ gamma-aminobutyric acid (GABA):** There is ↓ expression of the enzyme necessary to create GABA in the hippocampus of schizophrenic patients.
- **↓ levels of glutamate receptors:** Schizophrenic patients have fewer NMDA receptors; this correlates with the psychotic symptoms observed with NMDA antagonists like ketamine.

Prognostic Factors

Forty to fifty percent of patients remain significantly impaired after their diagnosis, while only 20–30% function fairly well in society with medication. About 50% of patients with schizophrenia attempt suicide. Several factors are associated with a better or worse prognosis:

Associated with Better Prognosis

- Later onset
- Good social support
- Positive symptoms
- Mood symptoms
- Acute onset
- Female sex
- Few relapses
- Good premorbid functioning

Associated with Worse Prognosis

- Early onset
- Poor social support
- Negative symptoms
- Family history
- Gradual onset
- Male sex
- Many relapses
- Poor premorbid functioning (social isolation, etc)
- Comorbid substance abuse

Treatment

A multimodality approach is the most effective, and therapy must be tailored to the needs of the specific patient. **Pharmacologic** treatment consists primarily of antipsychotic medications, otherwise known as neuroleptics. (For more detail, see Psychopharmacology chapter.)

- **First-generation antipsychotic medications:** *Chlorpromazine, thioridazine, trifluoperazine, haloperidol.* These are dopamine (mostly D_2) antagonists.
  - More effective against positive symptoms with minimal impact on negative symptoms.
  - Common side effects include extrapyramidal symptoms, neuroleptic malignant syndrome, and tardive dyskinesia (see below).

- **Second-generation antipsychotic medications:** *Risperidone, clozapine, olanzapine, quetiapine, aripiprazole, ziprosidone.*
  - These antagonize serotonin receptors (5-HT_2) as well as dopamine receptors.
  - Originally believed to be more effective than older antipsychotic medications, current research has shown no significant difference between the two groups in treating negative symptoms.
  - They have a much lower incidence of extrapyramidal side effects, but are now known to ↑ the risk for metabolic syndrome.
  - Medications should be taken for at least 4 weeks before efficacy is determined.
  - Typically, clozapine is reserved for patients who have failed multiple antipsychotic trials due to its ↑ risk of agranulocytosis.

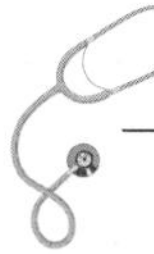

Schizophrenic patients who are treated with *second-generation* (atypical) antipsychotic medications need a careful medical evaluation for **metabolic syndrome.** This includes checking waist circumference, body mass index (BMI), fasting blood glucose, lipid assessment, and blood pressure.

Behavioral therapy attempts to improve patients' ability to function in society. Patients are helped through a variety of methods to improve their social skills, become self-sufficient, and minimize disruptive behaviors. **Family therapy** and **group therapy** are also useful adjuncts.

IMPORTANT SIDE EFFECTS AND SEQUELAE OF ANTIPSYCHOTIC MEDICATIONS

Side effects of antipsychotic medications include:

1. Extrapyramidal symptoms (especially with the use of high-potency traditional antipsychotics):
   - Dystonia (spasms) of face, neck, and tongue
   - Parkinsonism (resting tremor, rigidity, bradykinesia)
   - Akathisia (feeling of restlessness)

   Treatment: Antiparkinsonian agents (benztropine, diphenhydramine, etc), benzodiazepines, beta-blockers (specifically indicated for akathisia)
2. Anticholinergic symptoms (especially low-potency traditional antipsychotics and atypical antipsychotics): Dry mouth, constipation, blurred vision.
   Treatment: As per symptom (eyedrops, stool softeners, etc)
3. Metabolic syndrome (second-generation antipsychotics): A constellation of conditions—↑ blood pressure, ↑ insulin levels, excess body fat around the waist or abnormal cholesterol levels—that occur together, ↑ the risk for developing cardiovascular disease, stroke, and type 2 diabetes.
   Treatment: Consider switching to a first-generation antipsychotic or a more "weight-neutral" second-generation antipsychotic such as aripiprazole or ziprasidone. Monitor lipids and blood glucose measurements. Refer the patient to primary care for appropriate treatment of hyperlipidemia, diabetes, etc. Encourage appropriate diet, exercise, and smoking cessation.
4. Tardive dyskinesia (high-potency antipsychotics): Darting or writhing movements of face, tongue, and head.
   Treatment: Discontinue or reduce the offending agent and consider substituting an atypical neuroleptic. Benzodiazepines, beta blockers, and cholinomimetics may be used short term. The movements often persist despite withdrawal of the offending drug. Although less common, atypical neuroleptics can cause tardive dyskinesia in some patients.
5. Neuroleptic malignant syndrome (high-potency antipsychotics):
   - Change in mental status, autonomic changes (high fever, elevated blood pressure, tachycardia), "lead pipe" rigidity, sweating, elevated

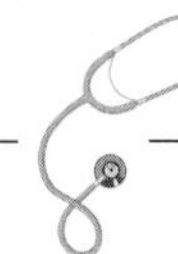

Patients who are treated with *first-generation* (typical) antipsychotic medication need to be closely monitored for **extrapyramidal symptoms,** such as acute dystonia and tardive dyskinesia.

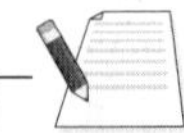

High-potency neuroleptics (such as haloperidol and trifluoperazine) have a higher incidence of extrapyramidal side effects, while *low-potency* neuroleptics (such as chlorpromazine and thioridazine) have primarily anticholinergic side effects.

creatine phosphokinase (CPK) levels, leukocytosis, and metabolic acidosis.

- A medical emergency that requires prompt withdrawal of all antipsychotic medications and immediate medical assessment and treatment.
- May be observed in any patient being treated with neuroleptic medications at any time but is more frequently associated with the initiation of treatment and at higher IV/IM dosing of high-potency neuroleptics.
- Patients with a history of prior neuroleptic malignant syndrome are at an ↑ risk of recurrent episodes when treated with neuroleptic agents.

6. Prolonged QT interval and other electrocardiogram changes, hyperprolactinemia (→ gynecomastia, galactorrhea, amenorrhea, diminished libido, and impotence), hematologic effects (agranulocytosis may occur with *clozapine*, necessitating weekly blood draws when this medication is used), ophthalmologic conditions (*thioridazine* may cause irreversible retinal pigmentation at high doses; deposits in lens and cornea may occur with *chlorpromazine*), dermatologic conditions (such as rashes and photosensitivity).

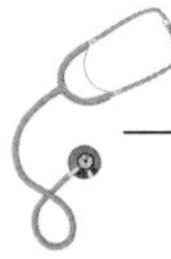

Tardive dyskinesia occurs most often in older women after at least 6 months of medication. Though 50% of patients will experience spontaneous remission, prompt discontinuation of the agent is important because the condition may become permanent.

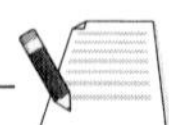

Beta blockers and digoxin are known to exacerbate psychosis in predisposed patients.

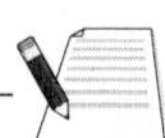

Up to 20% of long-term hospitalized patients treated with antipsychotics end up suffering from tardive dyskinesia.

SCHIZOPHRENIFORM DISORDER

Diagnosis and DSM-IV Criteria

The diagnosis of schizophreniform disorder is made using the same DSM-IV criteria as schizophrenia. The only difference between the two is that in schizophreniform disorder the symptoms have lasted between 1 and 6 months, whereas in schizophrenia the symptoms must be present for > 6 months.

Prognosis

One-third of patients recover completely; two-thirds progress to schizoaffective disorder or schizophrenia.

Treatment

Hospitalization, 3- to 6-month course of antipsychotics, and supportive psychotherapy.

SCHIZOAFFECTIVE DISORDER

Diagnosis and DSM-IV Criteria

The diagnosis of schizoaffective disorder is made in patients who:

- Meet criteria for either major depressive episode, manic episode, or mixed episode (during which criteria for schizophrenia are also met).
- Have had delusions or hallucinations for 2 weeks in the absence of mood disorder symptoms (this condition is necessary to differentiate schizoaffective disorder from mood disorder with psychotic features).
- Have mood symptoms present for substantial portion of psychotic illness.
- Have symptoms not due to general medical condition or drugs.

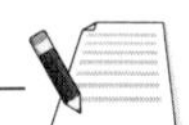

If a schizophrenia presentation has not been present for 6 months, think *schizophreniform disorder.*

PROGNOSIS

Approximately 60–80% will progress to schizophrenia.

TREATMENT

- Hospitalization and supportive psychotherapy.
- Medical therapy: Antipsychotics and mood stabilizers; antidepressants or electroconvulsive therapy (ECT) may be indicated for treatment of mood symptoms.

BRIEF PSYCHOTIC DISORDER

DIAGNOSIS AND DSM-IV CRITERIA

Patient with psychotic symptoms as defined for schizophrenia; however, the symptoms last from 1 day to 1 month. Symptoms must not be due to general medical condition or drugs. This is a rare diagnosis, much less common than schizophrenia. May be seen in reaction to extreme stress such as bereavement, sexual assault, etc.

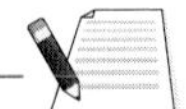

> Patients with borderline personality disorder may have transient, stress-related psychotic experiences. These are considered part of their underlying Axis II disorder and not diagnosed as a brief psychotic disorder.

PROGNOSIS

There is a 50–80% recovery rate; 20–50% may eventually be diagnosed with schizophrenia or mood disorder.

TREATMENT

Brief hospitalization, supportive psychotherapy, course of antipsychotics for psychosis itself, and/or benzodiazepines for agitation.

DELUSIONAL DISORDER

Delusional disorder occurs more often in older patients (after age 40), immigrants, and the hearing impaired.

DIAGNOSIS AND DSM-IV CRITERIA

To be diagnosed with delusional disorder, the following criteria must be met (see Table 2-1):

- Nonbizarre, fixed delusions for at least 1 month.
- Does not meet criteria for schizophrenia.
- Functioning in life not significantly impaired.

TYPES OF DELUSIONS

Patients are further categorized based on the types of delusions they experience:

- **Erotomanic type:** Delusion revolves around love (Eros is the goddess of love).
- **Grandiose type:** Inflated self-worth.
- **Somatic type:** Physical delusions.
- **Persecutory type:** Delusions of being persecuted.
- **Jealous type:** Delusions of unfaithfulness.
- **Mixed type:** More than one of the above.

TABLE 2-1. Schizophrenia vs. Delusional Disorder

Schizophrenia	Delusional Disorder

▪ Bizarre delusions (or nonbizarre)
▪ Daily functioning significantly impaired
▪ Must have two or more of the following:
  ▪ Delusions
  ▪ Hallucinations
  ▪ Disorganized speech
  ▪ Disorganized behavior
  ▪ Negative symptoms
	▪ Nonbizarre delusions (never bizarre)
	▪ Daily functioning not significantly impaired
	▪ Does not meet the criteria for schizophrenia as described in left column

Prognosis

- 50%: Full recovery
- 20%: ↓ symptoms
- 30%: No change

Treatment

Very difficult to treat. Psychotherapy may be helpful. Antipsychotic medications are often ineffective, but a course of them should be tried (usually a high-potency traditional antipsychotic or one of the newer atypical antipsychotics is used).

SHARED PSYCHOTIC DISORDER

Diagnosis and DSM-IV Criteria

Also known as *folie à deux*, shared psychotic disorder is diagnosed when a patient develops the same delusional symptoms as someone he or she is in a close relationship with. Most people suffering from shared psychotic disorder are family members.

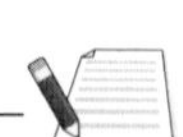

Folie à deux, also known as induced psychotic disorder (IPD), involves delusions or hallucinations that are transmitted from one individual to another.

Prognosis

Twenty to forty percent will recover upon removal from the inducing person.

Treatment

- The most important treatment step is to separate the patient from the person who is the source of shared delusions (usually a family member with an underlying psychotic disorder).
- Psychotherapy should be undertaken, and antipsychotic medications should be used if symptoms have not improved in 1–2 weeks after separation.

CULTURE-SPECIFIC PSYCHOSES

These are psychoses seen only within certain cultures:

	Psychotic Manifestation	Culture
Koro	Patient believes that his penis is shrinking and will disappear causing his death.	Asia
Amok	Sudden unprovoked outbursts of violence of which the person has no recollection. Person often commits suicide afterward.	Malaysia, Southeast Asia
Brain fag	Headache, fatigue, and visual disturbances in male students.	Africa

COMPARING TIME COURSES AND PROGNOSES OF PSYCHOTIC DISORDERS

Time Course

- < 1 month—brief psychotic disorder
- 1–6 months—schizophreniform disorder
- > 6 months—schizophrenia

SchizophreniFORM = the FORMation of a schizophrenic, but not quite there (ie, < 6 months).

Prognosis from Best to Worst

Mood disorder > brief psychotic disorder > schizoaffective disorder > schizophreniform disorder > schizophrenia.

QUICK AND EASY DISTINGUISHING FEATURES

- **Schizophrenia:** Lifelong psychotic disorder.
- **Schizophreniform:** Schizophrenia for < 6 months.
- **Schizoaffective:** Schizophrenia + mood disorder.
- **Schizotypal** (personality disorder): Paranoid, odd or magical beliefs, eccentric, lack of friends, social anxiety. Criteria for true psychosis are not met.
- **Schizoid** (personality disorder): Withdrawn, lack of enjoyment from social interactions, emotionally restricted.

NOTES

HIGH-YIELD FACTS IN

Mood Disorders

MOOD DISORDERS

Mood disorders often have chronic courses that are marked by relapses with relatively normal functioning between episodes. Like most psychiatric diagnoses, mood episodes may be triggered by a medical condition or drug (prescribed or illicit). Always investigate medical or substance-induced causes (see below) before making a diagnosis.

Differential Diagnosis of Mood Disorders Secondary to General Medical Conditions

Medical Causes of a Depressive Episode

Cerebrovascular disease (stroke, myocardial infarction)
Endocrinopathies (diabetes mellitus, Cushing syndrome, Addison disease, hypoglycemia, hyper/hypothyroidism, hyper/hypocalcemia)
Parkinson disease
Viral illnesses (eg, mononucleosis)
Carcinoid syndrome
Cancer (especially lymphoma and pancreatic carcinoma)
Collagen vascular disease (eg, systemic lupus erythematosus)

Medical Causes of a Manic Episode

Metabolic (hyperthyroidism)
Neurological disorders (temporal lobe seizures, multiple sclerosis)
Neoplasms
HIV infection

Mood Disorders Secondary to Medication or Substance Use

Medication/Substance-Induced Depressive Episodes

EtOH
Antihypertensives
Barbiturates
Corticosteroids
Levodopa
Sedative-hypnotics
Anticonvulsants
Antipsychotics
Diuretics
Sulfonamides
Withdrawal from psychostimulants (eg, cocaine, amphetamines)

Medication/Substance-Induced Mania

Antidepressants
Sympathomimetics
Dopamine
Corticosteroids
Levodopa
Bronchodilators

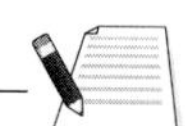

Stroke patients are at very high risk for developing depression.

MAJOR DEPRESSIVE DISORDER (MDD)

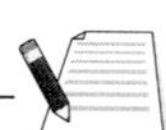

Major depressive disorder has the highest rate of suicide of any disorder.

MDD is marked by episodes of depressed mood associated with loss of interest in daily activities. Patients may be unaware of their depressed mood or may express vague, somatic complaints (fatigue, headache, abdominal pain, muscle tension, etc).

DIAGNOSIS AND DSM-IV CRITERIA

- At least one major depressive episode (see above).
- No history of manic or hypomanic episode.

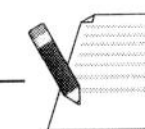

Most adults with clinically significant depression never see a mental health professional but often see a primary care physician for other reasons.

EPIDEMIOLOGY

- Lifetime prevalence: 16.2% in the United States (48 million Americans).
- Onset at any age, but average age of onset is 40.
- Twice as prevalent in women than men during reproductive years. Prevalence is equal between men and women after menopause and before menses.
- No ethnic or socioeconomic differences.
- Prevalence in elderly from 25 to 50%.
- Depression can ↑ mortality for patients with other comorbidities (diabetes, cardiovascular disease).

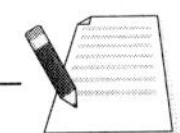

Anhedonia is the inability to experience pleasure, which is a common finding in depression.

SLEEP PROBLEMS ASSOCIATED WITH MDD

- Multiple awakenings.
- Initial and terminal insomnia (hard to fall asleep and early morning awakenings).
- Hypersomnia (excessive sleepiness).
- Rapid eye movement (REM) sleep shifted to earlier in night and stages 3 and 4 ↓.

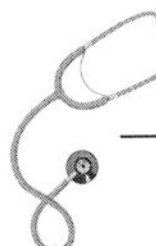

The two most common kinds of sleep disturbances associated with depression are difficulty falling asleep and early morning awakening.

ETIOLOGY

The exact cause of depression is unknown, but biological, genetic, environmental, and psychosocial factors each contribute.

- The leading theory is that depression is caused by neurotransmitter deficiencies in the brain. ↓ brain and cerebrospinal fluid (CSF) levels of serotonin and its main metabolite, 5-hydroxyindolacetic acid (5-HIAA), are found in depressed patients.
- Abnormal regulation of beta-adrenergic receptors has also been shown.
- Drugs that ↑ availability of serotonin, norepinephrine, and dopamine often alleviate symptoms of depression.
- **High cortisol:** Hyperactivity of hypothalamic-pituitary-adrenal axis as shown by failure to suppress cortisol levels in dexamethasone suppression test.
- **Abnormal thyroid axis:** Thyroid disorders are associated with depressive symptoms.
- Gamma-aminobutyric acid (GABA) and endogenous opiates may have a role.
- **Psychosocial/life events:** Stable family and social functioning have been shown to be good prognostic indicators in the course of major depression.
- **Genetics:** First-degree relatives are two to three times more likely to have MDD. Concordance rate for monozygotic twins is about 50–70%, and 10–25% for dizygotic twins.

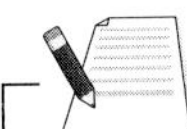

The Hamilton Rating Score is the standard measure of depression severity that is used in research to assess the effectiveness of therapies.

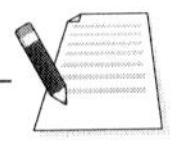

Loss of a parent before age 11 is associated with the later development of major depression.

COURSE AND PROGNOSIS

- If left untreated, depressive episodes are self-limiting but usually last from 6 to 13 months. Generally, episodes occur more frequently as the disorder progresses. The risk of a subsequent major depressive episode is

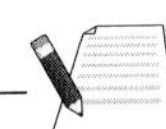

Pancreatic cancer has a high association with depression.

Unique Types and Features of Depressive Disorders

- **Melancholic:** Forty to sixty percent of hospitalized patients with major depression. Characterized by anhedonia, early morning awakenings, psychomotor disturbance, excessive guilt, and anorexia. For example, you may diagnose "major depressive disorder with melancholic features."
- **Atypical:** Characterized by hypersomnia, hyperphagia, reactive mood, leaden paralysis, and hypersensitivity to interpersonal rejection.
- **Catatonic:** Features include catalepsy (immobility), purposeless motor activity, extreme negativism or mutism, bizarre postures, and echolalia. Especially responsive to ECT. May also be applied to bipolar disorder.
- **Psychotic:** Ten to twenty-five percent of hospitalized depressions. Characterized by the presence of delusions or hallucinations.

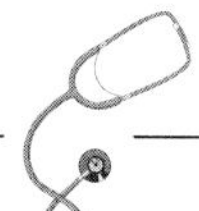

The catatonic type of major depression is usually treated with antidepressants and antipsychotics concurrently.

BEREAVEMENT

Bereavement, also known as simple grief, is a reaction to a major loss, usually of a person. Symptoms often last for 2 months and include crying spells, problems sleeping, and trouble concentrating at work. Normal bereavement should not include gross disorganization or suicidality.

It is important to differentiate bereavement from psychiatric disorders (major depression, acute stress disorder, adjustment disorder).

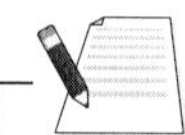

Kübler-Ross model of grief consists of five stages:

1. Denial
2. Anger
3. Bargaining
4. Depression
5. Acceptance

Normal Grief Versus Depression

In normal grief, illusions are common but suicidal thoughts are rare and symptoms usually last < 2 months. Mild cognitive disorder typically lasts < 1 year and patients can be treated with mild benzodiazepines for sleep.

In depression, however, hallucinations and delusions are common, suicidal thoughts may be present, and symptoms generally persist > 2 months. Mild cognitive disorder usually lasts for > 1 year and patients can be treated with antidepressants, mood stabilizers, or ECT.

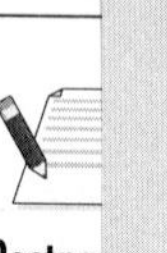

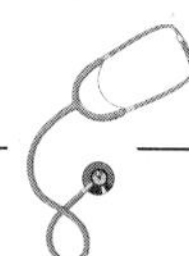

Bipolar I disorder may have **psychotic features** (delusions or hallucinations); these can occur during major depressive *or* manic episodes. Always remember to include bipolar disorder in your differential of a psychotic patient.

BIPOLAR I DISORDER

Bipolar I disorder involves episodes of mania and of major depression; however, episodes of major depression are *not* required for the diagnosis. It is traditionally known as **manic depression.**

Diagnosis and DSM-IV Criteria

The only requirement for this diagnosis is the occurrence of one manic or mixed episode (10–20% of patients experience only manic episodes). Between manic episodes, there may be interspersed euthymia, major depressive episodes, dysthymia, or hypomanic episodes, but none of these are required for diagnosis.

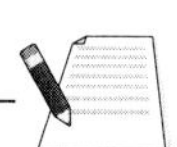

Rapid cycling is defined by the occurrence of four or more mood episodes in 1 year (major depressive, manic, mixed, etc).

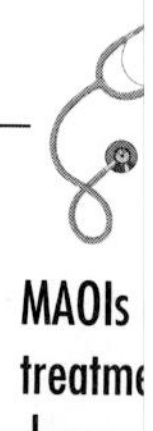

Epidemiology

- Lifetime prevalence: 1%.
- Women and men are equally affected.
- No ethnic differences seen.
- Onset usually before age 30.
- Frequently misdiagnosed and thereby mistreated.

Etiology

- Biological, environmental, psychosocial, and genetic factors are all important.
- First-degree relatives of patients with bipolar disorder are 8–18 times more likely to develop the illness.
- Concordance rates for monozygotic twins are approximately 40–70%, and rates for dizygotic twins are 5–25%.
- Bipolar I has the highest genetic link of all major psychiatric disorders.

Course and Prognosis

- Untreated manic episodes generally last about 3 months.
- The course is usually chronic with relapses; as the disease progresses, episodes may occur more frequently.
- Ninety percent of individuals after one manic episode will have a repeat manic episode within 5 years.
- Bipolar disorder has a worse prognosis than MDD.
- Lithium prophylaxis between episodes helps to ↓ the risk of relapse.
- Twenty-five to fifty percent of people with bipolar disorder attempt suicide, and 15% die by suicide, which are significantly higher rates than that of MDD.

Treatment

- **Pharmacotherapy:**
  - Lithium is a mood stabilizer; 70% treated with lithium show partial reduction of mania. Long-term use reduces suicide risk. Mortality rate is 25% from acute overdose, due to low therapeutic index.
  - Anticonvulsants (carbamazepine or valproic acid) are also mood stabilizers. They are especially useful for rapid cycling bipolar disorder and mixed episodes, although associated with ↑ risk of suicide.
  - Atypical antipsychotics (olanzapine, quetiapine, ziprasidone) are effective as both monotherapy and adjunct therapy for acute mania, with careful monitoring of adverse effects.
  - Antidepressants are discouraged as monotherapy due to concerns of activating mania or hypomania. The addition of antidepressants as adjunctive therapy to mood stabilizers has not shown to be effective.
- **Psychotherapy:** Supportive psychotherapy, family therapy, group therapy (prolongs remission once the acute manic episode has been controlled).
- **ECT:**
  - Works well in treatment of manic episodes.
  - Usually requires more treatments than for depression.
  - Especially effective for refractory or life-threatening acute mania or depression.

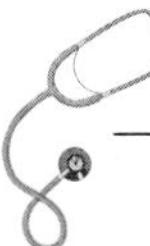

Side effects of lithium include:

- Weight gain
- Tremor
- Gastrointestinal disturbances
- Fatigue
- Cardiac arrhythmias
- Seizures
- Goiter/hypothyroidism
- Leukocytosis (benign)
- Coma
- Polyuria (nephrogenic diabetes insipidus)
- Polydipsia
- Alopecia
- Metallic taste

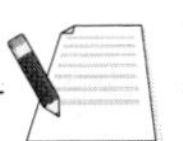

ECT is the best treatment for a manic woman in pregnancy. It provides a good alternative to antipsychotics and can be used with relative safety in all trimesters.

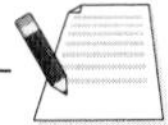

Treatment for bipolar disorder includes lithium, carbamazepine (for rapid cyclers), and valproic acid.

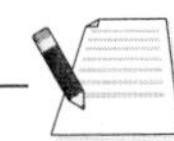

A patient with a history of postpartum mania should be treated with antidepressants and lithium in subsequent pregnancies as prophylaxis. However, these are relative contraindications to breast-feeding.

BIPOLAR II DISORDER

Alternatively called **recurrent major depressive episodes with hypomania.**

DIAGNOSIS AND DSM-IV CRITERIA

History of one or more major depressive episodes and at least one **hypomanic** episode. *Remember*: If there has been a full manic episode *even in the past*, then the diagnosis is *not* bipolar II disorder, but bipolar I.

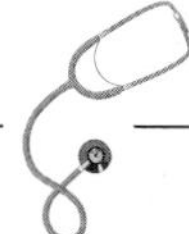

Symptoms of dysthymic disorder—

CHASES

Poor **C**oncentration or difficulty making decisions
Feelings of **H**opelessness
Poor **A**ppetite or overeating
In**S**omnia or hypersomnia
Low **E**nergy or fatigue
Low **S**elf-esteem

EPIDEMIOLOGY

- More prevalent than bipolar I.
- Slightly more common in women.
- Onset usually before age 30.
- No ethnic differences seen.
- Frequently misdiagnosed as unipolar depression and thereby mistreated.

ETIOLOGY

Same as bipolar I disorder (see above).

COURSE AND PROGNOSIS

Tends to be chronic, requiring long-term treatment.

TREATMENT

More prevalent than bipolar I but fewer studies focus on the treatment for bipolar II. Thus, until further studies, treatment is the same as bipolar I disorder (see above).

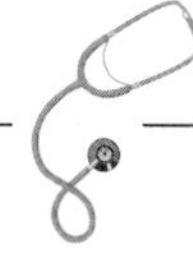

MDD tends to be episodic, while dysthymic disorder is generally persistent.

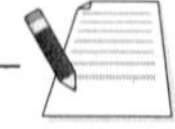

Dysthymic disorder (DD) = 2 D's
2 years of depression
2 listed criteria
Never asymptomatic for > **2** months

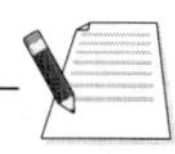

Double depression: Patients with major depressive disorder with dysthymic disorder during residual periods.

DYSTHYMIC DISORDER

Patients with dysthymic disorder have chronic, mild depression most of the time with no discrete episodes. They rarely need hospitalization.

DIAGNOSIS AND DSM-IV CRITERIA

1. Depressed mood for the majority of time most days for at least 2 years (in children or adolescents for at least 1 year)
2. At least two of the following:
   - Poor concentration or difficulty making decisions
   - Feelings of hopelessness
   - Poor appetite or overeating
   - Insomnia or hypersomnia
   - Low energy or fatigue
   - Low self-esteem
3. During the 2-year period:
   - The person has not been without the above symptoms for > 2 months at a time.
   - No major depressive episode.
   - The patient must never have had a manic or hypomanic episode (this would make the diagnosis bipolar disorder or cyclothymic disorder, respectively).

EPIDEMIOLOGY

- Lifetime prevalence: 6%.
- Two to three times more common in women.
- Onset before age 25 in 50% of patients.

COURSE AND PROGNOSIS

Twenty percent of patients will develop major depression, 20% will develop bipolar disorder, and > 25% will have lifelong symptoms.

TREATMENT

- Cognitive therapy and insight-oriented psychotherapy are most effective.
- Antidepressant medications (SSRIs, TCAs, or MAOIs) are useful when used concurrently with psychotherapy.

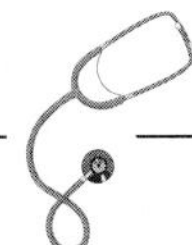

Dysthymia can never have psychotic features. If a patient has delusions or hallucinations with "depression," consider another diagnosis (eg, major depression with psychotic features, schizoaffective, etc).

CYCLOTHYMIC DISORDER

Alternating periods of hypomania and periods with mild to moderate depressive symptoms.

DIAGNOSIS AND DSM-IV CRITERIA

- Numerous periods with hypomanic symptoms and periods with depressive symptoms for at least 2 years.
- The person must never have been symptom free for > 2 months during those 2 years.
- No history of major depressive episode or manic episode.

EPIDEMIOLOGY

- Lifetime prevalence: < 1%.
- May coexist with borderline personality disorder.
- Onset usually age 15–25.
- Occurs equally in males and females.

COURSE AND PROGNOSIS

Chronic course; one-third of patients are eventually diagnosed with bipolar disorder.

TREATMENT

Antimanic agents as used to treat bipolar disorder (see above).

OTHER DISORDERS OF MOOD IN DSM-IV

- Minor depressive disorder: Episodes of two to four depressive symptoms that do not meet the full five or more criteria for major depressive disorder; euthymic periods are also seen, unlike in dysthymic disorder. Still associated with significant functional impairments, and 18% may fit the criteria for MDD within 1 year.
- Recurrent brief depressive disorder.
- Premenstrual dysphoric disorder.
- Mood disorder due to a general medical condition.

- Substance-induced mood disorder.
- Mood disorder not otherwise specified (NOS).

SPECIFIERS OF MOOD DISORDERS IN DSM-IV

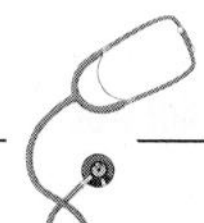

> Triad for seasonal affective disorder:
> - Irritability
> - Carbohydrate craving
> - Hypersomnia

Specifiers are not considered a separate mood disorder but rather a subtype within any major mood disorder.

- Seasonal affective disorder (SAD): At least 2 consecutive years of two major depressive episodes during the same season, most commonly the winter but may occur in any season. Patients with fall-onset SAD ("winter depression") often respond to light therapy.
- Postpartum major depression (PMD): Onset within 4 weeks of delivery.

ADJUSTMENT DISORDERS

Adjustment disorders occur when maladaptive behavioral or emotional symptoms develop after a stressful life event. Symptoms begin within 3 months after the event, end within 6 months, and cause significant impairment in daily functioning or interpersonal relationships.

Diagnosis and DSM-IV Criteria

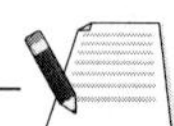

> In adjustment disorder, the stressful event is not life threatening (such as a divorce, death of a loved one, or loss of a job). In posttraumatic stress disorder (PTSD), it is.

1. Development of emotional or behavioral symptoms within 3 months after a stressful life event. These symptoms produce either:
   - Severe distress in excess of what would be expected after such an event
   - Significant impairment in daily functioning
2. The symptoms are not those of bereavement.
3. Symptoms resolve within 6 months after stressor has terminated.

Subtypes: Symptoms are coded based on a predominance of either depressed mood, anxiety, disturbance of conduct (such as aggression), or combinations of the above.

Epidemiology

- Adjustment disorders are very common.
- They occur twice as often in females.
- They are most frequently diagnosed in adolescents but may occur at any age.

Etiology

Triggered by psychosocial factors.

Prognosis

May be chronic if the stressor is recurrent; symptoms resolve within 6 months of cessation of stressor (by definition).

Treatment

- Supportive psychotherapy (most effective)
- Group therapy
- Pharmacotherapy for associated symptoms (insomnia, anxiety, or depression)

HIGH-YIELD FACTS IN

Anxiety and Adjustment Disorders

TABLE 4-1. Symptoms of Anxiety

Cardiac	Palpitations, tachycardia, hypertension
Pulmonary	Shortness of breath, choking sensation
Neurologic	Dizziness, light-headedness, hyperreflexia, mydriasis (pupil dilation), tremors, tingling in the peripheral extremities
Psychological	Restlessness (pacing), "butterflies in the stomach"
Other	Sweating, gastrointestinal, urinary urgency and frequency

Anxiety is the subjective experience of fear and its physical manifestations. It is a common, normal response to a perceived threat. It is important for clinicians to be able to distinguish normal (see Table 4-1) from pathological anxiety.

Pathological anxiety is inappropriate (there is either no real source of fear or the source is not sufficient to account for the severity of the symptoms). In people with anxiety disorders, the **symptoms interfere with daily functioning** and interpersonal relationships.

- Anxiety disorders are caused by a combination of genetic, environmental, biological (see Table 4-2), and psychosocial factors.
- Associated with neurotransmitter imbalances, including ↑ activity of norepinephrine and ↓ activity of gamma-aminobutyric acid (GABA) and serotonin.

TABLE 4-2. Biological Causes of Anxiety

Medical Causes of Anxiety Disorders	Medication- or Substance-Induced Anxiety Disorders
Hyperthyroidism	Caffeine intake and withdrawal Theophylline
Vitamin B_{12} deficiency	Amphetamines
Hypoxia	Alcohol and sedative withdrawal
Neurological disorders (epilepsy, brain tumors, multiple sclerosis, cerebrovascular disease, etc)	Other illicit drug withdrawal
	Mercury or arsenic toxicity
	Organophosphate or benzene toxicity
Cardiovascular disease	Penicillin
Anemia	Sulfonamides
Pheochromocytoma	Sympathomimetics
Hypoglycemia	Antidepressants

- Lifetime prevalence: Women 30%, men 19%.
- Develop more frequently in higher socioeconomic groups.
- Types of anxiety disorders include:
  - Panic disorder
  - Agoraphobia
  - Specific and social phobias
  - Obsessive-compulsive disorder
  - Posttraumatic stress disorder
  - Acute stress disorder
  - Generalized anxiety disorder
  - Anxiety disorder secondary to general medical condition
  - Substance-induced anxiety disorder

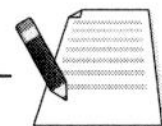

Panic attack criteria—PANICS
Palpitations
Abdominal distress
Numbness, nausea
Intense fear of death
Choking, chills, chest pain
Sweating, shaking, shortness of breath

PANIC ATTACKS

Panic attacks are discrete periods of heightened anxiety and fear that classically occur in patients with panic disorder, but can also be seen with other anxiety disorders (phobic disorders, posttraumatic stress disorder).

Panic attacks peak within 10 minutes and usually last < 25 minutes. They may be provoked by triggers or come on spontaneously. To diagnose a panic attack, a patient must have at least four of the following symptoms: palpitations, sweating, shaking, shortness of breath, choking sensation, chest pain, nausea or abdominal distress, light-headedness, depersonalization (feeling detached from oneself) or derealization (feeling out of reality), fear of losing control or "going crazy," fear of dying, numbness or tingling, chills or hot flushes.

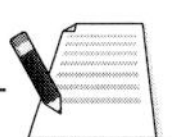

Panic attacks are associated with conditions such as mitral valve prolapse, asthma, pulmonary embolus, angina, and anaphylaxis.

A patient's first panic attack is usually unexpected by the patient, but it may follow a period of stress or physical exertion. Subsequent attacks usually occur spontaneously but may be associated with specific situations.

PANIC DISORDER

Panic disorder is characterized by spontaneous recurrent panic attacks with no obvious precipitant. Patients with panic disorder suffer from panic attacks on average two times per week but may range from several times per day to a few times per year. They usually last between 20 and 30 minutes, and anticipatory anxiety about having another attack is common between episodes.

Diagnosis and DSM-IV Criteria

- To qualify for panic disorder, at least one of the attacks must be followed by a minimum of 1 month of the following:
  - Persistent concern about having additional attacks
  - Worry about the implications of the attack (losing control or "going crazy")
  - A significant change in behavior related to the attacks (avoidance of situations that may provoke attacks)
- There is a vast differential diagnosis for panic disorder, and it is important to rule out other conditions before making the diagnosis of panic disorder (Table 4-3).
- Always specify whether panic disorder is **with agoraphobia** or **without agoraphobia** (see below).

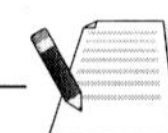

More than 40% of patients presenting with chest pain and normal angiograms may have panic disorder.

TABLE 4-3. Differential Diagnosis of Panic Attacks/Disorder

Medical	Congestive heart failure, angina, myocardial infarction, thyrotoxicosis, temporal lobe epilepsy, multiple sclerosis, pheochromocytoma, carcinoid syndrome, chronic obstructive pulmonary disease (COPD)
Medications/drugs	Amphetamine, caffeine, nicotine, cocaine, and hallucinogen intoxication; alcohol or opiate withdrawal
Other psychiatric disorders commonly associated with panic disorder	Depressive disorders, phobic disorders, obsessive-compulsive disorder, and posttraumatic stress disorder

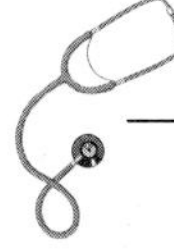

A classic example of panic disorder would be a female who repeatedly visits the ER with episodes of a racing heart, sweating, shortness of breath, and a fear of "going crazy" or of dying.

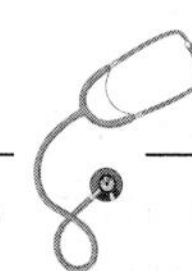

Always start SSRIs at low dose and ↑ slowly in panic disorder patients because some SSRIs can have side effects that may initially worsen anxiety.

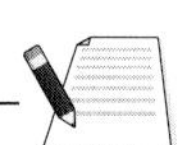

Characteristic situations avoided in agoraphobia include bridges, crowds, buses, trains, or any open areas outside the home.

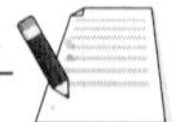

Common Specific Phobias

- Fear of animals
- Fear of heights
- Fear of blood or needles
- Fear of illness or injury
- Fear of death
- Fear of flying

Etiology

- Biological, genetic, and psychosocial factors contribute to the development of panic disorder.
- Associated with dysregulation of the autonomic nervous system, central nervous system, and cerebral blood flow.
- Related to changes in neurotransmitter activity (↑ activity of norepinephrine, ↓ activity of serotonin and GABA).
- Panic attacks may be induced by: caffeine, nicotine, hyperventilation.

Epidemiology

- Lifetime prevalence: 2–5%.
- Two to three times more common in females than males.
- Strong genetic component: Four to eight times greater risk of panic disorder if first-degree relative is affected.
- Onset usually from late teens to early thirties (average age 25), but may occur at any age.

Course and Prognosis

Panic disorder has a variable course but is often chronic. Relapses are common with discontinuation of medical therapy:

- Ten to twenty percent of patients continue to have significant symptoms that interfere with daily functioning.
- Fifty percent continue to have mild, infrequent symptoms.
- Thirty to forty percent remain free of symptoms after treatment.

Treatment

- Best long-term treatment is selective serotonin reuptake inhibitors (SSRIs), especially paroxetine and sertraline (typically take 2–4 weeks to become effective, and higher doses are required than for depression).
- Other antidepressants (clomipramine, imipramine) may also be used.
- Benzodiazepines are effective immediately but are best used temporarily because of their risk of causing tolerance and dependency.
- Treatment should continue for at least 8–12 months, as relapse is common after discontinuation of therapy.
- *Nonpharmacological treatments:* Relaxation training, biofeedback, cognitive therapy, insight-oriented psychotherapy.

AGORAPHOBIA

Agoraphobia is the fear of being alone in public places.

- The anxiety → the avoidance of being in places or situations from which escape or help might be difficult.
- It often develops secondary to panic attacks due to apprehension about having subsequent attacks in public places where escape may be difficult.
- It can be diagnosed alone or as panic disorder with agoraphobia (50–75% of patients have coexisting panic disorder).
- When a coexisting panic disorder is treated, agoraphobia usually resolves.
- When agoraphobia is not associated with panic disorder, it is usually chronic and debilitating.

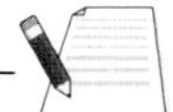

Common Social Phobias
- Speaking in public
- Eating in public
- Using public restrooms

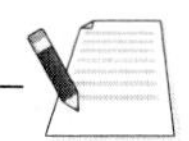

For a person with issues of shyness, the provoked anxiety has to interfere with their daily functioning for the diagnosis to be consider social phobia.

SPECIFIC PHOBIAS AND SOCIAL PHOBIA

A phobia is defined as an irrational fear that → avoidance of the feared object or situation. A *specific phobia* is a strong, exaggerated fear of a specific object or situation; a *social phobia* (also called **social anxiety disorder**) is a fear of social situations in which embarrassment can occur.

DIAGNOSIS AND DSM-IV CRITERIA

The diagnostic criteria for **specific phobias** are as follows:

1. Persistent excessive fear brought on by a specific situation or object.
2. Exposure to the situation brings about an immediate anxiety response.
3. Patient recognizes that the fear is excessive.
4. The situation is avoided when possible or tolerated with intense anxiety.
5. If person is under age 18, duration must be at least 6 months.

The diagnosis of **social phobia** has the same criteria as above except that the feared situation is related to social settings in which the patient might be embarrassed or humiliated in front of other people.

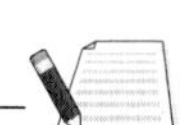

Substance disorders, especially alcohol dependence, are often comorbid in phobic patients. Up to one-third of phobic patients also have associated major depression.

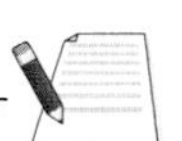

Performance anxiety is often successfully treated with beta blockers.

EPIDEMIOLOGY

- Phobias are the **most common mental disorders** in the United States.
- At least 5–10% of the population is afflicted with a phobic disorder.
- The diagnosis of specific phobia is more common than social phobia.
- Onset can be as early as 5 years old for phobias such as seeing blood, and as old as 35 for situational fears (such as a fear of heights).
- The average age of onset for social phobias is mid-teens.
- Women are two times as likely to have specific phobia as men.
- Social phobia occurs equally in men and women.

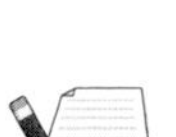

Systemic desensitization is the gradual exposure of a patient to the feared object or situation while teaching relaxation and breathing techniques. The opposite, ***flooding***, would be directly confronting the patient with their full fear.

ETIOLOGY

The cause of phobias is most likely multifactorial, with genetic and neurochemical factors playing a role.

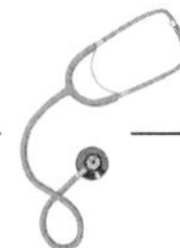

Treatment of OCD often requires *higher doses* of SSRIs than treatment of depression.

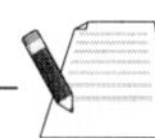

The diagnostic criteria for posttraumatic stress disorder (PTSD) requires the presence of a traumatic experience, persistent avoidance, hyperarousal (or ↑ psychological and/or physiological tension), and reexperiencing the traumatic event—all for more than a month.

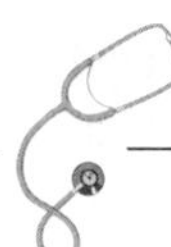

A patient who is experiencing recurrent thoughts and nightmares about a past trauma should be screened for PTSD.

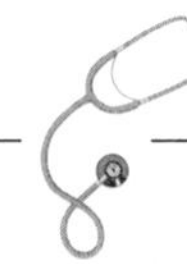

Cognitive processing therapy is a modified form of cognitive-behavioral therapy in which thoughts, feelings, and meanings of the event are revisited and questioned.

POSTTRAUMATIC STRESS DISORDER (PTSD)

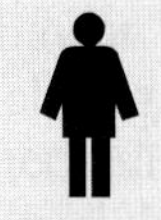

A 26-year-old man is brought in by his girlfriend for frequent nightmares, persistent symptoms of anxiety, and insomnia for the past 3 months. She reports that he is usually social and extroverted but lately has been withdrawn and unwilling to engage much. Upon further questioning, she mentions that he was in a car accident several months prior in which he sustained minor injuries but witnessed his brother die. *Diagnosis?* PTSD. These symptoms must be present for at least a month.

PTSD is a response to a catastrophic (life-threatening) life experience in which the patient reexperiences the trauma, avoids reminders of the event, and experiences emotional numbing or hyperarousal.

DIAGNOSIS AND DSM-IV CRITERIA

- Patient has experienced or witnessed a traumatic event (eg, war, rape, or natural disaster).
- The event was potentially harmful or fatal, and the initial reaction was intense fear or horror.
- Persistent reexperiencing of the event (eg, in dreams, flashbacks, recurrent recollections, or intense psychological distress to cues that relate to the traumatic event).
- Avoidance of stimuli associated with the trauma (eg, avoiding a location that will remind him or her of the event or having difficulty recalling details of the event).
- Numbing of responsiveness (limited range of affect, feelings of detachment or estrangement from others, etc).
- Persistent symptoms of ↑ arousal (eg, difficulty sleeping, outbursts of anger, hypervigilance, exaggerated startle response, or difficulty concentrating).
- Symptoms must be present for at least 1 month.

COMORBIDITIES

Patients have a high incidence of associated substance abuse and depression.

PROGNOSIS

One-half of patients remain symptom free after 3 months of treatment.

TREATMENT

- **Pharmacological:**
  - Antidepressants: SSRIs, TCAs (imipramine, doxepin), monoamine oxidase inhibitors (MAOIs)
  - Anticonvulsants (for flashbacks and nightmares)
- **Other:**
  - Therapy: Cognitive-behavioral, supportive, psychodynamic
  - Relaxation training
  - Support groups, family therapy
  - Eye movement desensitization and reprocessing (EMDR)

TABLE 4-4. PTSD Versus Acute Stress Disorder

PTSD	ACUTE STRESS DISORDER
Event occurred at any time in past	Event occurred < 1 month ago
Symptoms last > 1 month	Symptoms last < 1 month

Addictive medications (benzodiazepines) should be avoided in the treatment of PTSD because of the high rate of substance abuse in these patients.

ACUTE STRESS DISORDER (ASD)

DIAGNOSIS AND DSM-IV CRITERIA

The diagnosis of ASD is reserved for patients who experience a major traumatic event but have anxiety symptoms for only a short duration. To qualify for this diagnosis, the symptoms must occur within 1 month of the trauma and last for a maximum of 1 month. Symptoms are similar to those of PTSD (see Table 4-4).

TREATMENT

Same as treatment for PTSD (see above).

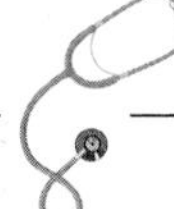

If a patient is exhibiting anxiety and dysfunction 2 weeks after watching his friend die in a car accident, he could qualify for acute stress disorder, but not PTSD until the symptoms have lasted > 1 month.

Mrs. Martin is a 24-year-old law student who arrives at the outpatient psychiatry clinic accompanied by her husband. She complains of difficulty falling asleep for which she requests sleep medication. She reports that she feels "stressed" about the number of readings she has to complete for school and frequently worries about failing her exams. She says, "I feel tired, I can't concentrate." She also complains of frequent headaches and associated muscle spasms that usually resolve with the use of naproxen. She adds that her husband keeps telling her to relax, and describes her as "a worrier." She asks that you speak to her husband, and he reports, "My wife is concerned about everything; she'll worry about me having an accident on the way home, about not getting the job she wants in the future, about not making enough money, the list goes on and on." Mrs. Martin reports that these symptoms have been present for many years but have worsened during the past 6 months, and she now finds it difficult to control her worries.

Mrs. Martin denies any other symptoms but reports a history of depression treated with antidepressants in the past. Family history reveals that her mother is treated for obsessive-compulsive disorder. A physical exam demonstrates tachycardia and sweating. Lab test results are pending.

What is Mrs. Martin's most likely diagnosis?

Her most likely diagnosis is generalized anxiety disorder (GAD). Mrs. Martin and her husband report that she has a history of worrying excessively about a number of events and activities in her life and has been unsuccessful in controlling these worries. She is also experiencing a sleep disturbance, fatigue, muscle tension, and a ↓ in concentration. The patient reports having suffered these symptoms for many years with worsening during the last six months. Patients with GAD commonly report somatic symptoms such as those described above (eg, tachycardia,

(continued)

sweating), however, a complete physical exam and medical workup should be performed in order to rule out medical conditions (eg, hyperthyroidism) or substance use. Also, remember GAD is frequently comorbid with other axis I disorders and a careful history should be undertaken to rule out depression.

What are Mrs. Martin's treatment options?

First-line pharmacological treatment for GAD includes the use of serotonin-norepinephrine reuptake inhibitors (SNRI; venlafaxine) and SSRIs. Other options include the use of benzodiazepines and buspirone. Cognitive-behavioral therapy (CBT) should also be undertaken, as studies routinely show that in patients with anxiety disorders, the combination of CBT with medication achieves better remission rates than either treatment alone.

GENERALIZED ANXIETY DISORDER (GAD)

Patients with GAD have persistent, excessive hyperarousal and anxiety about general daily events. They usually first seek out a nonpsychiatrist specialist because of their somatic complaints, such as muscle tension or fatigue.

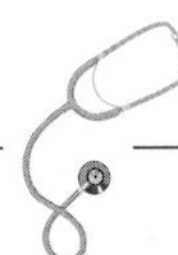

When diagnosing GAD, make sure to rule out medical conditions that produce anxiety states such as hyperthyroidism. Ask about caffeine intake.

Diagnosis of GAD requires at least 6 months of three out of six symptoms.

Diagnosis and DSM-IV Criteria

- Excessive anxiety and worry about daily events and activities (that is difficult to control) for at least 6 months.
- Must be associated with at least three of the following: restlessness, fatigue, difficulty concentrating, irritability, muscle tension, sleep disturbance.

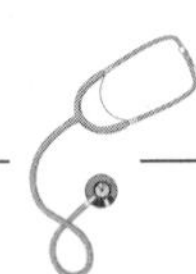

If a patient complains of constant worries about multiple areas of his life, it must cause significant distress, occur most days of the week, and last for > 6 months to qualify as GAD.

Epidemiology

- GAD is very common in the general population (lifetime prevalence: 45%).
- Women are two times as likely to have GAD as men.
- Onset is usually before the age of 20.
- Fifty to ninety percent of patients with GAD have a coexisting mental disorder, especially major depression, social or specific phobia, or panic disorder.

Etiology

Not completely understood, but biological and psychosocial factors contribute.

Prognosis

GAD is chronic, with lifelong, fluctuating symptoms in 50% of patients. The other half of patients will fully recover within several years of therapy.

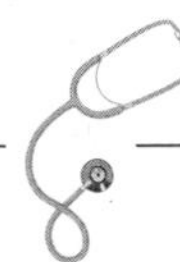

In GAD, the anxiety is *free-floating,* as opposed to being fixed on a specific person, event, or activity.

Treatment

The most effective treatment approach is a combination of psychotherapy (cognitive-behavioral therapy) and pharmacotherapy:

- Antidepessants (SSRIs, buspirone, venlafaxine).
- If benzodiazepines (clonazepam, diazepam) are used, they should be tapered off when possible because of risk of tolerance and dependence.

sun

HIGH-YIELD FACTS IN

Personality Disorders

DEFINITION

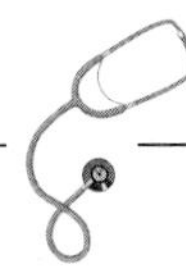

Many people have odd tendencies and quirks; these are not pathological unless they cause significant distress or impairment in daily functioning.

Personality is one's set of stable, predictable emotional and behavioral traits. Personality *disorders* involve deeply ingrained, inflexible patterns of relating to others that are **maladaptive** and cause significant impairment in social or occupational functioning. The disorders include marked limitations in problem solving and low stress tolerance. Patients with personality disorders lack insight about their problems; their symptoms are either **ego-syntonic** or viewed as immutable. They have a rigid view of themselves and others and around their fixed patterns have little insight. Patients with personality disorders are vulnerable to developing symptoms of Axis I disorders during stress.

Personality disorders are Axis II diagnoses.

DIAGNOSIS AND DSM-IV CRITERIA

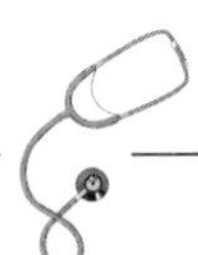

Personality disorder criteria—

CAPRI

Cognition
Affect
Personal **R**elations
Impulse control

1. Pattern of behavior/inner experience that deviates from the person's culture and is manifested in two or more of the following ways:
   - Cognition
   - Affect
   - Personal relations
   - Impulse control
2. The pattern:
   - Is **pervasive** and **inflexible** in a broad range of situations
   - Is **stable** and has an onset no later than adolescence or early adulthood
   - → significant distress in functioning
   - Is not accounted for by another mental/medical illness or by use of a substance

The international prevalence of personality disorders is 6%. Personality disorders vary by gender. Many patients with personality disorders will meet the criteria for more than one disorder. They should be classified as having all of the disorders for which they qualify.

CLUSTERS

Personality disorders are divided into three clusters:

- **Cluster A**—schizoid, schizotypal, and paranoid:
  - Patients seem eccentric, peculiar, or withdrawn.
  - Familial association with psychotic disorders.
- **Cluster B**—antisocial, borderline, histrionic, and narcissistic:
  - Patients seem emotional, dramatic, or inconsistent.
  - Familial association with mood disorders.
- **Cluster C**—avoidant, dependent, and obsessive-compulsive:
  - Patients seem anxious or fearful.
  - Familial association with anxiety disorders.

Personality disorder not otherwise specified (NOS) includes disorders that do not fit into cluster A, B, or C (including passive-aggressive personality disorder and depressive personality disorder).

Etiology

- Biological, genetic, and psychosocial factors during childhood and adolescence contribute to the development of personality disorders.
- The prevalence of personality disorders in monozygotic twins is several times higher than in dizygotic twins.

Treatment

- Personality disorders are generally very difficult to treat, especially since few patients are aware that they need help. The disorders tend to be chronic and lifelong.
- In general, pharmacologic treatment has limited usefulness (see individual exceptions below) except in treating coexisting symptoms of depression, anxiety, and the like.
- Psychotherapy and group therapy are usually the most helpful.

Cluster A

These patients are perceived as eccentric or hermetic by others and can have symptoms that meet criteria for psychosis (Table 5-1).

Paranoid Personality Disorder (PPD)

Patients with PPD have a pervasive distrust and suspiciousness of others and often interpret motives as malevolent. They tend to blame their own problems on others and seem angry and hostile. They are often characterized as being pathologically jealous, which leads them to think that their sexual partners or spouses are cheating on them.

TABLE 5-1. Cluster A Personality Disorders and Classic Clinical Examples

Personality Disorder	Clinical Example
Paranoid personality disorder	A 30-year-old man says his wife has been cheating on him because he does not have a good enough job to provide for her needs. He also claims that on his previous job, his boss laid him off because he did a better job than his boss. Refuses couples therapy because he believes the treater will side with his wife. Believes neighbors are critical of him.
Schizoid personality disorder	A 45-year-old scientist works in the lab most of the day and has no friends, according to his coworkers. Has not been able to keep his job because of failure to collaborate with others. He expresses no desire to make friends and is content with his single life. He has no evidence of a thought disorder.
Schizotypal personality disorder	A 35-year-old man dresses in a space suit every Tuesday and Thursday. He has computers set up in his basement to "detect the precise time of alien invasion." He has no evidence of auditory or visual hallucinations.

Diagnosis and DSM-IV Criteria

- Diagnosis requires a general distrust of others, beginning by early adulthood and present in a variety of contexts.
- At least four of the following must also be present:
  1. Suspicion (without evidence) that others are exploiting or deceiving him or her.
  2. Preoccupation with doubts of loyalty or trustworthiness of acquaintances.
  3. Reluctance to confide in others.
  4. Interpretation of benign remarks as threatening or demeaning.
  5. Persistence of grudges.
  6. Perception of attacks on his or her character that are not apparent to others; quick to counterattack.
  7. Recurrence of suspicions regarding fidelity of spouse or lover.

Epidemiology

- Prevalence: 0.5 to 2.5%.
- Prevalence is higher in men than in women.
- Higher incidence in family members of schizophrenics.
- The disorder is misdiagnosed in minority groups, immigrants, and deaf people.

Differential Diagnosis

- *Paranoid schizophrenia:* Unlike patients with schizophrenia, patients with paranoid personality disorder *do not have any fixed delusions and are not frankly psychotic*, although they may have transient psychosis under stressful situations.
- *Social disenfranchisement and social isolation:* Without a social support system, persons can react with suspicion to others. The differential in favor of the diagnosis can be made by the assessment of others in close contact with the person, who identify what they consider as excess suspicion, etc.

Course and Prognosis

- Some patients with PPD may eventually be diagnosed with schizophrenia.
- The disorder usually has a chronic course, causing lifelong marital and job-related problems.

Treatment

- Psychotherapy is the treatment of choice.
- Patients may also benefit from antianxiety medications or short course of antipsychotics for transient psychosis.

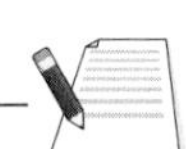

Unlike with avoidant personality disorder, patients with schizoid personality disorder *prefer* to be alone.

Schizoid Personality Disorder

Patients with schizoid personality disorder have a lifelong pattern of social withdrawal. They are often perceived as eccentric and reclusive. They are quiet and unsociable and have a constricted affect. They have *no desire for close relationships* and prefer to be alone.

Diagnosis and DSM-IV Criteria

- A pattern of voluntary social withdrawal and restricted range of emotional expression, beginning by early adulthood and present in a variety of contexts.
- Four or more of the following must also be present:
  1. Neither enjoying nor desiring close relationships (including family)
  2. Generally choosing solitary activities
  3. Little (if any) interest in sexual activity with another person
  4. Taking pleasure in few activities (if any)
  5. Few close friends or confidants (if any)
  6. Indifference to praise or criticism
  7. Emotional coldness, detachment, or flattened affect

Epidemiology

- Prevalence: Approximately 7%.
- Prevalence in men is twice that of women.

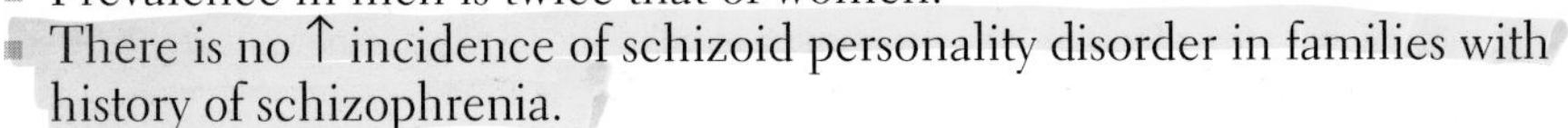

- There is no ↑ incidence of schizoid personality disorder in families with history of schizophrenia.

Differential Diagnosis

- *Paranoid schizophrenia*: Unlike patients with schizophrenia, patients with schizoid personality disorder do not have any fixed delusions, although these may exist transiently in some patients.
- *Schizotypal personality disorder*: Patients with schizoid personality disorder do not have the same eccentric behavior or magical thinking seen in patients with schizotypal personality disorder. Schizotypal patients are more similar to schizophrenic patients in terms of odd perception, thought, and behavior.

Course

Usually chronic course, but not always lifelong.

Treatment

Similar to paranoid personality disorder:

- Psychotherapy is the treatment of choice; group therapy is often beneficial.
- Low-dose antipsychotics (short course) if transiently psychotic, or antidepressants if comorbid major depression is diagnosed.

Schizotypal Personality Disorder

Patients with schizotypal personality disorder have a pervasive pattern of eccentric behavior and peculiar thought patterns. They are often perceived as strange and eccentric. The disorder was developed out of the observation that certain family traits predominate in first-degree relatives with schizophrenia.

Diagnosis and DSM-IV Criteria

- A pattern of social deficits marked by eccentric behavior, cognitive or perceptual distortions, and discomfort with close relationships, beginning by early adulthood and present in a variety of contexts.
- Five or more of the following must be present:
  1. Ideas of reference (excluding delusions of reference)
  2. Odd beliefs or magical thinking, inconsistent with cultural norms

TABLE 5-2. Cluster B Personality Disorders and Classic Clinical Examples

Personality Disorder	Clinical Example
Antisocial personality disorder	A 30-year-old unemployed man has been accused of killing three senior citizens after robbing them. He is surprisingly charming in the interview. In his adolescence, he was arrested several times for stealing cars and assaulting other kids.
Borderline personality disorder	A 23-year-old medical student attempted to slit her wrist because things did not work out with a man she had been dating over the past 3 weeks. She states that guys are jerks and "not worth her time." She often feels that she is "alone in this world."
Histrionic personality disorder	A 33-year-old scantily clad woman comes to your office complaining that her fever feels like "she is burning in hell." She vividly describes how the fever has affected her work as a teacher.
Narcissistic personality disorder	A 48-year-old company CEO is rushed to the ED after an automobile accident. He does not let the residents operate on him and requests the chief of trauma surgery because he is "vital to the company." He makes several business phone calls in the ED to stay on "top of his game."

3. Unusual perceptual experiences (such as bodily illusions)
4. Suspiciousness
5. Inappropriate or restricted affect
6. Odd or eccentric appearance or behavior
7. Few close friends or confidants
8. Odd thinking or speech (vague, stereotyped, etc)
9. Excessive social anxiety

- Magical thinking may include:
  - Belief in clairvoyance or telepathy
  - Bizarre fantasies or preoccupations
  - Belief in superstitions
- Odd behaviors may include involvement in cults or strange religious practices.

Epidemiology

Prevalence: 3.0%.

Differential Diagnosis

- *Paranoid schizophrenia:* Unlike patients with schizophrenia, patients with schizotypal personality disorder are not frankly psychotic (though they can become transiently so under stress), nor do they have fixed delusions.
- *Schizoid personality disorder*: Patients with schizoid personality disorder do not have the same eccentric behavior seen in patients with schizotypal personality disorder.

Course

- Course is chronic or patients may eventually develop schizophrenia.
- Premormid personality type for a patient with schizophrenia.

Treatment

- Psychotherapy is the treatment of choice to help develop social skills training.
- Short course of low-dose antipsychotics if necessary (for transient psychosis). Antipsychotics may help decrease social anxiety and suspicion in interpersonal relationships.

Cluster B

Includes antisocial, borderline, histrionic, and narcissistic personality disorders. These patients are often emotional, impulsive, and dramatic (Table 5-2).

Mr. Harris is a 35-year-old man with no prior psychiatric history who was arrested for assaulting his pregnant girlfriend. While in jail, he reports feeling depressed, and you are called in for a psychiatric evaluation. Mr. Harris is cooperative during the evaluation and presents as friendly and likeable. He reports that he is innocent of his charges and expresses feeling sad and tearful since his incarceration 2 days ago. He requests that you transfer him to the mental health unit at the correctional facility. However, you perform a thorough evaluation, and you do not find symptoms suggestive of a mood or psychotic disorder. When asked if he has been incarcerated before, he reports a history of multiple arrests and convictions for robbery and gun possession. He reports that he is unemployed because he has been "in and out of jail" during the past 5 years. He provides explanations of his limited involvement in these past crimes and does not appear remorseful.

Mr. Harris reveals a pattern of repeated fights since childhood and says that he quit school while in the ninth grade after being suspended for smoking pot on school grounds. Mr. Harris reports that throughout his childhood he bullied others, and laughs when recounting an episode during which he threw his cat against the wall to see it bounce back. He denies any family history of psychiatric illnesses, but reports that his father is currently incarcerated for drug trafficking.

What is his Axis II diagnosis?

Mr. Harris's diagnosis is antisocial personality disorder. His history shows a pervasive pattern of disregard for and violation of others since age 15, and there is evidence of conduct disorder with onset before age 15 years. Remember that, although it is common, not all criminals have antisocial personality disorder.

What are some associated findings?

Antisocial personality disorder is more prevalent in males, is associated with low socioeconomic background, and has a genetic predisposition. It has been found that the children of parents with antisocial personality disorder have an ↑ risk for this disorder, somatization disorder, and substance-related disorders.

ANTISOCIAL PERSONALITY DISORDER

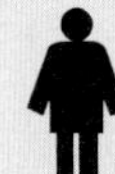

A 26-year-old man has a history of multiple criminal arrests and is the son of two alcoholic parents. His brother recalls him setting their pet dog on fire as a kid. *Think: antisocial personality disorder.*

Antisocial personality disorder is a disorder in which a person violates the rights of others without showing guilt. Men, especially those with alcoholic parents, are more likely than women to have this condition.

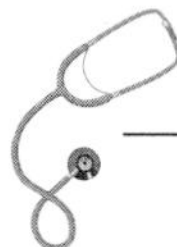

Symptoms of antisocial personality disorder—CONDUCT

Capraciousness
Oppressive
Non-confrontational
Deceitful
Unlawful
Carefree
Temper

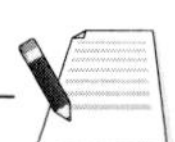

Antisocial personality disorder begins in childhood as **conduct disorder.** Patient may have a history of being abused (physically or sexually) as a child or a history of hurting animals or starting fires. It is often associated with violations of the law.

Patients diagnosed with antisocial personality disorder show superficial conformity to social norms but are exploitive of others and break rules to meet their own needs. Lack empathy and compassion; lack remorse for their actions. They are impulsive, deceitful, and often violate the law. They are skilled at reading social cues and appear charming and normal to others who meet them for the first time and do not know their history.

DIAGNOSIS AND DSM-IV CRITERIA

- Pattern of disregard for others and violation of the rights of others since age 15.
- Patients must be **at least 18 years old** for this diagnosis; history of behavior as a child/adolescent must be consistent with **conduct disorder** (see chapter on Psychiatric Disorders in Children).
- Three or more of the following should be present:
  1. Failure to conform to social norms by committing unlawful acts
  2. Deceitfulness/repeated lying/manipulating others for personal gain
  3. Impulsivity/failure to plan ahead
  4. Irritability and aggressiveness/repeated fights or assaults
  5. Recklessness and disregard for safety of self or others
  6. Irresponsibility/failure to sustain work or honor financial obligations
  7. Lack of remorse for actions

EPIDEMIOLOGY

- Prevalence: 3% in men and 1% in women.
- There is a higher incidence in poor urban areas and in prisoners but no racial difference.
- Genetic component: Five times ↑ risk among first-degree relatives.

DIFFERENTIAL DIAGNOSIS

Drug abuse: It is necessary to ascertain which came first. Patients who began abusing drugs before their antisocial behavior started may have behavior attributable to the effects of their addiction.

COURSE

- Usually has a chronic course, but some improvement of symptoms may occur as the patient ages.
- Many patients have multiple somatic complaints, and coexistence of substance abuse and/or major depression is common.
- There is ↑ morbidity from substance abuse, trauma, suicide, or homicide.

TREATMENT

- Psychotherapy is generally ineffective; dialectical behavior therapy (DBT) and behavioral therapy best choice.
- Pharmacotherapy may be used to treat symptoms of anxiety or depression, but use caution due to high addictive potential of these patients.

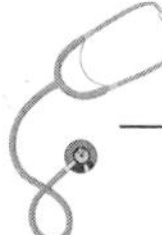

Symptoms of borderline personality disorder— IMPULSIVE

Impulsive
Moody
Paranoid under stress
Unstable self-image
Labile, intense relationships
Suicidal
Inappropriate anger
Vulnerable to abandonment
Emptiness

BORDERLINE PERSONALITY DISORDER (BPD)

Patients with BPD have unstable moods, behaviors, and interpersonal relationships. They fear abandonment and have poorly formed identity. Relationships begin with intense attachments and end with the slightest conflict. Aggression is common. They are impulsive and may have a history of repeated suicide attempts/gestures or episodes of self-mutilation. They have higher rates of childhood physical, emotional, and sexual abuse than the general population (25–35% of these patents report no such abuse).

DIAGNOSIS AND DSM-IV CRITERIA

- Pervasive pattern of impulsivity and unstable relationships, affects, self-image, and behaviors, present by early adulthood and in a variety of contexts.
- At least five of the following must be present:
  1. Desperate efforts to avoid real or imagined abandonment
  2. Unstable, intense interpersonal relationships (eg, extreme love-hate relationships)
  3. Unstable self-image
  4. Impulsivity in at least two potentially harmful ways (spending, sexual activity, substance use, binge eating, etc)
  5. Recurrent suicidal threats or attempts or self-mutilation
  6. Unstable mood/affect
  7. General feeling of emptiness
  8. Difficulty controlling anger
  9. Transient, stress-related paranoid ideation or dissociative symptoms

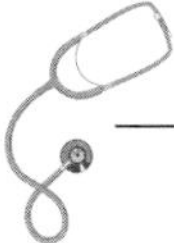

Borderline patients commonly use defense mechanism of *splitting*—they view others as all good or all bad. (Clinical example: "You are the only doctor who has ever helped me. Every doctor I met before you was horrible.")

EPIDEMIOLOGY

- Prevalence: 1–2%.
- Prevalence is twice as high in women than men.
- Suicide rate: 10%.

DIFFERENTIAL DIAGNOSIS

- *Schizophrenia*: Unlike patients with schizophrenia, patients with BPD do not have frank psychosis (may have transient psychosis, however, if decompensate under stress).
- *Bipolar II*: Mood swings experienced in BPD are moment-to-moment reactions to perceived environmental triggers. They also are not characterized by spending excess amounts of money or heightened sexual activity.

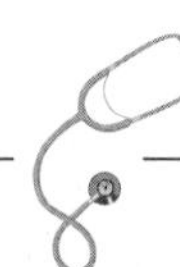

Pharmacotherapy has been shown to be more useful in BPD than in any other personality disorder.

COURSE

- Usually has a stable, chronic course.
- High incidence of coexisting major depression and/or substance abuse.
- ↑ risk of suicide (often because patients will make suicide gestures and kill themselves by accident).

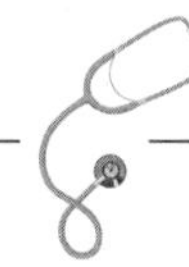

The name *borderline* comes from the patient's being on the borderline of neurosis and psychosis.

Treatment

- Psychotherapy (DBT) is the treatment of choice—behavior therapy, cognitive therapy, social skills training, etc.
- Pharmacotherapy to treat psychotic or depressive symptoms as necessary.

Histrionic Personality Disorder (HPD)

Patients with HPD exhibit attention-seeking behavior and excessive emotionality. They are dramatic, flamboyant, and extroverted but are unable to form long-lasting, meaningful relationships. They are often sexually inappropriate and provocative.

Diagnosis and DSM-IV Criteria

- Pattern of excessive emotionality and attention seeking, present by early adulthood and in a variety of contexts.
- At least five of the following must be present:
  1. Uncomfortable when not the center of attention
  2. Inappropriately seductive or provocative behavior
  3. Uses physical appearance to draw attention to self
  4. Has speech that is impressionistic and lacking in detail
  5. Theatrical and exaggerated expression of emotion
  6. Easily influenced by others or situation
  7. Perceives relationships as more intimate than they actually are

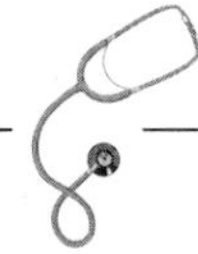

Histrionic patients often use defense mechanism of *regression*—they revert to childlike behaviors.

Epidemiology

- Prevalence: 2–3%.
- Women are more likely to have HPD than men.

Differential Diagnosis

Borderline personality disorder: Patients with BPD are more likely to suffer from depression, brief psychotic episodes, and to attempt suicide. HPD patients are generally more functional.

Course

Usually has a chronic course, with some improvement of symptoms with age.

Treatment

- Psychotherapy is the treatment of choice.
- Pharmacotherapy to treat associated depressive or anxious symptoms as necessary.

Narcissistic Personality Disorder (NPD)

Patients with NPD have a sense of superiority, a need for admiration, and a lack of empathy. They consider themselves "special" and will exploit others for their own gain. Despite their grandiosity, however, these patients often have fragile self-esteem.

Diagnosis and DSM-IV Criteria

- Pattern of grandiosity, need for admiration, and lack of empathy beginning by early adulthood and present in a variety of contexts.

- Five or more of the following must be present:
  1. Exaggerated sense of self-importance
  2. Preoccupation with fantasies of unlimited money, success, brilliance, etc
  3. Believes that he or she is "special" or unique and can associate only with other high-status individuals
  4. Needs excessive admiration
  5. Has sense of entitlement
  6. Takes advantage of others for self-gain
  7. Lacks empathy
  8. Envious of others or believes others are envious of him or her
  9. Arrogant or haughty

> Narcissism is characterized by an inflated sense of entitlement. People with narcissistic personality are often "fishing for compliments" and become irritated and anxious when they are not at the center of attention.

EPIDEMIOLOGY

Prevalence: < 1%.

DIFFERENTIAL DIAGNOSIS

Antisocial personality disorder: Both types of patients exploit others, but NPD patients want status and recognition, while antisocial patients want material gain or simply the subjugation of others. Narcissistic patients become depressed when they don't get the recognition they think they deserve.

COURSE

Usually has a chronic course; higher incidence of depression and midlife crises since these patients put such a high value on youth and power.

TREATMENT

- Psychotherapy is the treatment of choice. Group therapy may help these patients learn empathy.
- Antidepressants or lithium may be used as needed (for mood swings if a comorbid mood disorder is diagnosed).

Cluster C

Includes avoidant, dependent, and obsessive-compulsive personality disorders. These patients appear anxious and fearful (Table 5-3).

AVOIDANT PERSONALITY DISORDER

Patients with avoidant personality disorder have a pervasive pattern of social inhibition and an intense fear of rejection. They will avoid situations in which they may be rejected. Their fear of rejection is so overwhelming that it affects all aspects of their lives. They avoid social interactions and seek jobs in which there is little interpersonal contact. These patients *desire* companionship but are extremely shy and easily injured.

> Social phobia is the most common phobia in avoidant personality disorder.

DIAGNOSIS AND DSM-IV CRITERIA

- A pattern of social inhibition, hypersensitivity, and feelings of inadequacy since early adulthood.
- At least four of the following must be present:
  1. Avoids occupation that involves interpersonal contact due to a fear of criticism and rejection
  2. Unwilling to interact unless certain of being liked

TABLE 5-3. Cluster C Personality Disorders and Classic Clinical Examples

Personality Disorder	Clinical Example
Avoidant personality disorder	A 30-year-old postal worker rarely goes out with her coworkers and often makes excuses when they ask her to join them because she is afraid they will not like her. She wishes to go out and meet new people but, according to her, she is too "shy."
Dependent personality disorder	A 40-year-old man who lives with his parents has trouble deciding on how to go about having his car fixed. He calls his father at work several times to ask very trivial things. He has been unemployed over the past 3 years.
Obsessive-compulsive personality disorder	A 40-year-old secretary has been recently fired because of her inability to prepare some work projects in time. According to her, they were not in the right format and she had to revise them six times, which led to the delay. This has happened before but she feels that she is not given enough time.

3. Cautious of interpersonal relationships
4. Preoccupied with being criticized or rejected in social situations
5. Inhibited in new social situations because he or she feels inadequate
6. Believes he or she is socially inept and inferior
7. Reluctant to engage in new activities for fear of embarrassment

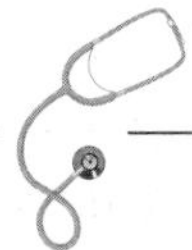

Symptoms of avoidant personality disorder—AFRAID

Avoids occupation with others
Fear of embarrassment and criticism
Reserved unless they are certain that they are liked
Always thinking rejection
Isolates from relationships
Distances self unless certain that they are liked

Epidemiology

- Prevalence: 1–10%.
- Sex ratio is not known.

Differential Diagnosis

- *Schizoid personality disorder:* Patients with avoidant personality disorder desire companionship but are extremely shy, whereas patients with schizoid personality disorder have no desire for companionship.
- *Social phobia (social anxiety disorder):* See chapter on Anxiety and Adjustment Disorders. Both disorders involve fear and avoidance of social situations. If the symptoms are an integral part of the patient's personality and have been evident since before adulthood, personality disorder is the more likely diagnosis. Social phobia involves a fear of *embarrassment* in a particular setting (speaking in public, urinating in public, etc), whereas avoidant personality disorder is an overall fear of *rejection* and a sense of inadequacy. However, a patient can have both disorders concurrently and should carry both diagnoses if criteria for each are met.
- *Dependent personality disorder:* Avoidant personality disorder patients cling to relationships, similar to dependent personality disorder patients; however, avoidant patients are slow to get involved, whereas dependents actively and aggressively seek relationships.

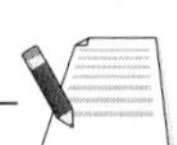

Schizoid patients *prefer* to be alone. Avoidant patients want to be with others but are too scared of rejection.

Course

- Course is usually chronic.
- Particularly difficult during adolescence, when attractiveness and socialization are important.

- ↑ incidence of associated anxiety and depressive disorders.
- If support system fails, patient is left very susceptible to depression, anxiety, and anger.

Treatment

- Psychotherapy, including assertiveness training, is most effective.
- Beta blockers may be used to control autonomic symptoms of anxiety, and selective serotonin reuptake inhibitors (SSRIs) may be prescribed for major depression.

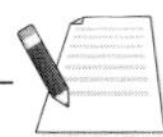

Regression is often seen in people with DPD. This is defined as going back to a younger age of maturity.

Dependent Personality Disorder (DPD)

Patients with DPD have poor self-confidence and fear separation. They have an excessive need to be taken care of and allow others to make decisions for them. They feel helpless when left alone.

Diagnosis and DSM-IV Criteria

- A pattern of submissive and clinging behavior due to excessive need to be taken care of.
- At least five of the following must be present:
  1. Difficulty making everyday decisions without reassurance from others
  2. Needs others to assume responsibilities for most areas of his or her life
  3. Cannot express disagreement because of fear of loss of approval
  4. Difficulty initiating projects because of lack of self-confidence
  5. Goes to excessive lengths to obtain support from others
  6. Feels helpless when alone
  7. Urgently seeks another relationship when one ends
  8. Preoccupied with fears of being left to take care of self

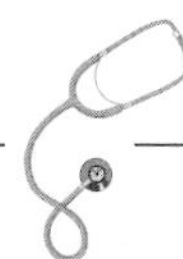

Symptoms of dependent personality disorder—

OBEDIENT

Obsessive about approval
Bound by others decisions
Enterprises are rarely initiated due to their lack of self-confidence
Difficult to make own decisions
Invalid feelings while alone
Engrossed with fears of self-reliance
Needs to be in a relationship
Tentative about decisions

Epidemiology

- Prevalence: Approximately 1%.
- Women are more likely to have DPD than men.

Differential Diagnosis

- *Avoidant personality disorder:* See discussion above.
- *Borderline and histrionic personality disorders:* Patients with DPD usually have a long-lasting relationship with one person on whom they are dependent. Patients with borderline and histrionic personality disorders are often dependent on other people, but they are unable to maintain a long-lasting relationship.

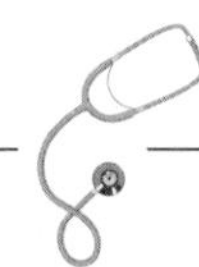

Many people with debilitating illnesses can develop dependent traits. However, to be diagnosed with DPD, the features must manifest in early adulthood.

Course

- Usually has a chronic course.
- Often, symptoms ↓ with age and/or therapy.
- Patients are prone to depression, particularly after loss of person on whom they are dependent.
- Difficulties with employment since they cannot act independently or without close supervision.

TREATMENT

- Psychotherapy, particularly groups and social skills training, is the treatment of choice.
- Pharmacotherapy may be used to treat associated symptoms of anxiety or depression.

OBSESSIVE-COMPULSIVE PERSONALITY DISORDER (OCPD)

Patients with OCPD have a pervasive pattern of perfectionism, inflexibility, and orderliness. They get so preoccupied with unimportant details that they are often unable to complete simple tasks in a timely fashion. They appear stiff, serious, and formal, with constricted affect. They are often successful professionally but have poor interpersonal skills.

DIAGNOSIS AND DSM-IV CRITERIA

- Pattern of preoccupation with orderliness, control, and perfectionism at the expense of efficiency, present by early adulthood and in a variety of contexts.
- At least four of the following must be present:
  1. Preoccupation with details, rules, lists, and organization such that the major point of the activity is lost
  2. Perfectionism that is detrimental to completion of task
  3. Excessive devotion to work
  4. Excessive conscientiousness and scrupulousness about morals and ethics
  5. Will not delegate tasks
  6. Unable to discard worthless objects
  7. Miserly
  8. Rigid and stubborn

EPIDEMIOLOGY

- Prevalence is unknown.
- Men are more likely to have OCPD than women.
- Occurs most often in the oldest child.
- ↑ incidence in first-degree relatives.

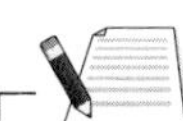

SSRIs often ↓ the invasive thoughts associated with OCD.

DIFFERENTIAL DIAGNOSIS

- *Obsessive-compulsive disorder (OCD)*: Patients with OCPD do not have the recurrent obsessions or compulsions that are present in obsessive-compulsive disorder. In addition, the symptoms of OCPD are **ego-syntonic** rather than ego-dystonic (as in OCD). That is, OCD patients are aware that they have a problem and wish that their thoughts and behaviors would go away.
- *Narcissistic personality disorder*: Both personalities involve assertiveness and achievement, but NPD patients are motivated by status, whereas OCD patients are motivated by the work itself.

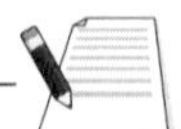

As the name suggests, OCD is characterized by obsession and compulsion. The obsession is the anxiety-producing thought aspect, while the compulsion is the behavioral aspect.

COURSE

- Unpredictable course.
- Some patients later develop obsessions or compulsions (OCD), some develop schizophrenia or major depressive disorder, and others may improve or remain stable.

TREATMENT

- Psychotherapy is the treatment of choice. Group therapy and behavior therapy may be useful.
- Pharmacotherapy may be used to treat associated symptoms as necessary.

Personality Disorder Not Otherwise Specified (NOS)

This diagnosis is reserved for personality disorders that do not fit into cluster A, B, or C. It includes passive-aggressive personality disorder, depressive personality disorder, sadomasochistic personality disorder, and sadistic personality disorder. Only passive-aggressive personality disorder and depressive personality disorder will be discussed below.

PASSIVE-AGGRESSIVE PERSONALITY DISORDER

Passive-aggressive personality disorder was once a separate personality disorder like those listed above but was relegated to the NOS category when DSM-IV was published. Patients with this disorder are stubborn, inefficient procrastinators. They alternate between compliance and defiance and passively resist fulfillment of tasks. They frequently make excuses for themselves and lack assertiveness. They attempt to manipulate others to do their chores, errands, and the like, and frequently complain about their own misfortunes. Psychotherapy is the treatment of choice.

DEPRESSIVE PERSONALITY DISORDER (DPD)

Persons with this disorder are characterized by lifelong traits of depressed-like state. These people are pessimistic, self-doubting, chronically unhappy, and distressed.

NOTES

HIGH-YIELD FACTS IN

Substance-Related Disorders

SUBSTANCE ABUSE/DEPENDENCE

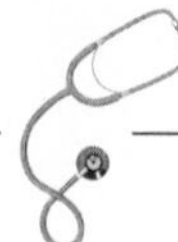

Substance abuse (need at least one)—

WILD

Work, school, or home role obligation failure
Interpersonal or social consequences
Legal problems
Dangerous use

DIAGNOSIS AND DSM-IV CRITERIA

Abuse is a pattern of substance use → impairment or distress for at least 12 months with one or more of the following manifestations:

1. Failure to fulfill obligations at work, school, or home
2. Use in dangerous situations (ie, driving a car)
3. Recurrent substance-related legal problems
4. Continued use despite social or interpersonal problems due to the substance use

Dependence is substance use → impairment or distress manifested by at least three of the following within a 12-month period:

1. Tolerance (see definition below)
2. Withdrawal (see definition below)
3. Using substance more than originally intended
4. Persistent desire or unsuccessful efforts to cut down on use
5. Significant time spent in getting, using, or recovering from substance
6. ↓ social, occupational, or recreational activities because of substance use
7. Continued use despite subsequent physical or psychological problem (eg, drinking despite worsening liver problems)

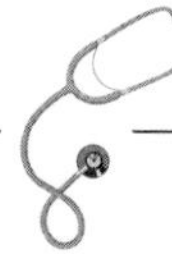

Note that it is possible to have substance dependence without having physiological dependence (ie, without having withdrawal or tolerance).

EPIDEMIOLOGY

- Lifetime prevalence of substance abuse or dependence in the United States is approximately 17%.
- More common in men than women.
- Alcohol and nicotine are the most commonly used substances.

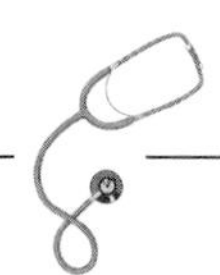

Substance-induced mood symptoms improve during abstinence, whereas *primary* mood symptoms persist.

PSYCHIATRIC SYMPTOMS

- Mood symptoms are common among persons with substance use disorders.
- Psychotic symptoms may occur with some substances.
- Personality disorders and psychiatric comorbidities (major depression, anxiety disorders) are common among persons with substance use disorders.
- It is often challenging to decide whether psychiatric symptoms are primary or substance induced.
- **Withdrawal:** The development of a substance-specific syndrome due to the cessation of substance use that has been heavy and prolonged.
- **Tolerance:** The need for ↑ amounts of the substance to achieve the desired effect *or* diminished effect if using the same amount of the substance.

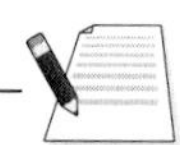

Withdrawal symptoms of a drug are usually opposite of its intoxication effects. For example, alcohol is sedating, but alcohol withdrawal can → brain excitation and seizures.

ACUTE INTOXICATION AND WITHDRAWAL

The intoxicated patient, or one experiencing withdrawal, can present several problems in both diagnosis and treatment. Since it is common for persons to abuse several drugs at once, the clinical presentation is often confusing, and signs/symptoms may be atypical. Always be on the lookout for polysubstance abuse.

Detection of Substance Abuse

See Table 6-1.

Treatment of Substance Abuse/Dependence

- Behavioral counseling should be part of every substance abuse/dependence treatment.
- Psychosocial treatments are effective and include motivational intervention (MI), cognitive-behavioral therapy (CBT), contingency management, and individual and group therapy.
- Twelve-step groups such as Alcoholics Anonymous (AA) and Narcotics Anonymous (NA) should also be encouraged as part of the treatment.
- Pharmacotherapy is available for some drugs of abuse, and will be discussed later in this chapter as relevant to a particular substance.

TABLE 6-1. Direct Testing for Substance Use

Alcohol	■ Stays in system for only a few hours. ■ Breathalyzer test, commonly used by police enforcement. ■ Blood/urine testing more accurate.
Cocaine	■ Urine drug screen positive for 2–4 days.
Amphetamines	■ Urine drug screen positive for 1–3 days. ■ Most assays are not of adequate sensitivity.
Phencyclidine (PCP)	■ Urine drug screen positive for 3–8 days. ■ Creatine phosphokinase (CPK) and aspartate aminotransferase (AST) are often elevated.
Sedative-hypnotics	In urine and blood for variable amounts of time. *Barbiturates:* ■ Short-acting (pentobarbital): 24 hours ■ Long-acting (phenobarbital): 3 weeks *Benzodiazepines:* ■ Short-acting (lorazepam): 3 days ■ Long-acting (diazepam): 30 days
Opioids	■ Urine drug test remains positive for 2–3 days, depending on opioid used. ■ Methadone and oxycodone will come up negative on a general screen (order a separate panel).
Marijuana	■ Urine detection: ■ In heavy users, up to 4 weeks (THC is released from adipose stores). ■ After a single use, about 3 days.

HIGH-YIELD FACTS

SUBSTANCE-RELATED DISORDERS

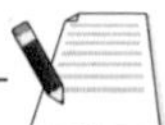

Pregnant women should not drink alcohol, as it can → fetal alcohol syndrome in the newborn, which is the leading cause of mental retardation in the United States.

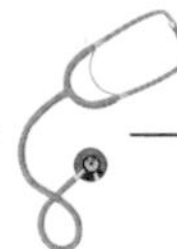

Alcohol is the most common co-ingestant in drug overdoses.

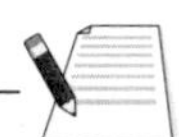

Most adults will show some signs of intoxication with BAL > 100 and obvious signs with BAL > 150 mg/dL.

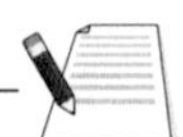

Ethanol, along with methanol and ethylene glycol, can be a cause of metabolic acidosis with ↑ anion gap.

Spousal abuse is more likely in homes in which male in involved in some kind of substance abuse, especially alcoholism.

ALCOHOL (ETOH)

- Alcohol activates gamma-aminobutyric acid (GABA) and serotonin receptors in the central nervous system (CNS), and inhibits glutamate receptors and voltage-gated calcium channels. GABA receptors are inhibitory, and glutamate receptors are excitatory. Thus, alcohol is a potent CNS depressant.
- Lifetime prevalence of alcohol dependence in the United States is 3–5% of women and 10% of men. Twice as many persons have met the diagnostic criteria for alcohol abuse during their lifetimes.
- Alcohol is metabolized in the following manner:
  1. Alcohol → acetaldehyde (enzyme: *alcohol dehydrogenase*).
  2. Acetaldehyde → acetic acid (enzyme: *aldehyde dehydrogenase*).

There is upregulation of these enzymes in heavy drinkers. Secondary to a gene variant, Asians often have less aldehyde dehydrogenase, resulting in flushing and nausea and protecting against alcohol dependence.

Intoxication

CLINICAL PRESENTATION

- The absorption and elimination rates of alcohol are variable and depend on many factors, including age, sex, body weight, chronic nature of use, duration of consumption, food in the stomach, and the state of nutrition and liver health.
- In addition to the above factors, the effects of EtOH also depend on the blood alcohol level (BAL). Serum EtOH level or an expired air breathalyzer can determine the extent of intoxication. As shown in Table 6-2, the effects/BAL may be ↓ if high tolerance has been developed.

TREATMENT

- **Monitor:** Airway, breathing, circulation, glucose, electrolytes, acid-base status.
- Give **thiamine** (to prevent or treat Wernicke's encephalopathy) and folate.
- **Naloxone** may be necessary to reverse effects of co-ingested opioids.
- A computed tomographic (CT) scan of the head may be necessary to rule out subdural hematoma or other brain injury.

TABLE 6-2. Clinical Presentation of Alcohol Intoxication

EFFECTS	BAL
↓ fine motor control	20–50 mg/dL
Impaired judgment and coordination	50–100 mg/dL
Ataxic gait and poor balance	100–150 mg/dL
Lethargy, difficulty sitting upright, difficulty with memory	150–250 mg/dL
Coma in the novice drinker	300 mg/dL
Respiratory depression, death possible	400 mg/dL

- Liver will eventually metabolize alcohol without any other interventions.
- Severely intoxicated patient may require mechanical ventilatory support with attention to acid-base balance, temperature, and electrolytes while he or she is recovering.
- Gastrointestinal evacuation (eg, gastric lavage, induction of emesis, and charcoal) is not indicated in the treatment of EtOH overdose unless a significant amount of EtOH was ingested within the preceding 30–60 minutes.

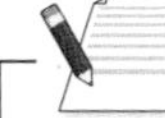

Alcohol is the most commonly abused substance in the US.

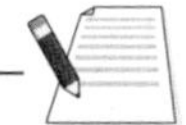

Attempted suicide is associated with mental illness, young females, and alcoholism.

Withdrawal

A 42-year-old man has routine surgery for a knee injury. After 72 hours in the hospital he becomes anxious, diaphoretic, and tachycardic. *What most likely can account for this patient's symptoms?* Alcohol withdrawal. *Treatment?* Benzodiazapine taper (chlordiazepoxide [Librium] is often considered the drug of choice). *What are you most concerned about?* Siezures, hypertension, and arrhythmias.

Chronic alcohol use has depressant effect on the CNS, and cessation of use causes a compensatory hyperactivity. Alcohol withdrawal is ***potentially lethal***!

Clinical Presentation

- Signs and symptoms of **alcohol withdrawal syndrome** include insomnia, anxiety, hand tremor, irritability, anorexia, nausea, vomiting, autonomic hyperactivity (diaphoresis, tachycardia, hypertension), psychomotor agitation, fever, seizures, hallucinations, and delirium (see Table 6-3).
- The earliest symptoms of EtOH withdrawal begin between 6 and 24 hours after the patient's last drink and depend on the duration and quantity of EtOH consumption.
- Generalized tonic-clonic **seizures** usually occur between 6 and 48 hours after cessation of drinking, with a peak around 13–24 hours.
- About a third of persons with seizures develop delirium tremens (DTs).
- Hypomagnesemia may predispose to seizures; thus, it should be corrected promptly.
- Seizures are treated with benzodiazepines. Long-term treatment with anticonvulsants is not recommended for alcohol withdrawal seizures.

TABLE 6-3. Alcohol Withdrawal Symptoms

EtOH withdrawal symptoms usually begin in 6–24 hours and last 2–7 days.
Mild: Irritability, tremor, insomnia. — 6 hours
Moderate: Diaphoresis, hypertension, tachycardia, fever, disorientation.
Severe: Tonic-clonic seizures, DTs, hallucinations.

Treat w/ long-acting benzo
diazepam
lorazepam
Chlordiazepoxide

Withdrawal seizures 12 - 48 hours
Alcoholic hallucinosis 12 - 24 hours
DT 48 - 96 hours

HIGH-YIELD FACTS

SUBSTANCE-RELATED DISORDERS

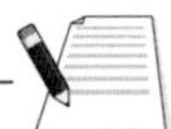

Delirium tremens carries a 15–25% mortality rate but occurs in only 5% of patients that are hospitalized for EtOH withdrawal.

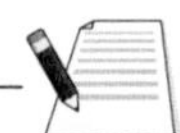

Confabulations, or memories of events that never occurred, are sometimes referred to as *false memories* and are often associated with Korsakoff's psychosis. Patients are unaware that they are "making these up."

DELIRIUM TREMENS (DTs)

- The most serious form of EtOH withdrawal.
- Usually begins 48–72 hours after the last drink but may occur later (90% of cases within 7 days).
- While only 5% of patients hospitalized for EtOH withdrawal develop DTs, there is a roughly 15–25% mortality rate if left untreated.
- Physical illness predisposes to the condition.
- Men develop DTs four to five times as often as women.
- In addition to delirium, symptoms of DTs may include hallucinations (most commonly visual), gross tremor, autonomic instability, and fluctuating levels of psychomotor activity.
- It is a medical emergency and should be treated with adequate doses of benzodiazepines.

TREATMENT

- Benzodiazepines (chlordiazepoxide, diazepam, or lorazepam) should be given in sufficient doses to keep the patient calm and lightly sedated, then tapered down slowly. Alternatively, carbamazepine, or valproic acid taper can be used.
- Antipsychotics and temporary restraints for severe agitation.
- Thiamine, folic acid, and a multivitamin to treat nutritional deficiencies ("banana bag").
- Electrolyte and fluid abnormalities must be corrected.
- Monitor withdrawal signs and symptoms with Clinical Institute Withdrawal Assessment (CIWA) scale.
- Careful attention must be given to the level of consciousness, and the possibility of trauma should be investigated.
- Check for signs of hepatic failure (eg, ascites, jaundice, caput medusae, coagulopathy).

Mr. Smith is a 42-year-old divorced man who arrives to the ED requesting treatment for alcohol detoxification. He reports that he began drinking at the age of 17 and that, although he initially drank only on the weekends, his alcohol use progressively increased to drinking half a pint of whiskey daily by the age of 35. At that time, he reports that he was referred to a 45-day inpatient alcohol abuse program after he arrived intoxicated at his workplace on several occasions, and was able to maintain his sobriety for 7 years. However, he reports that 2 years ago he relapsed into alcohol use after he divorced and was laid off from work due to "the economy."

Mr. Smith is currently living with his older sister and states that his drinking is "out of control." He had a DUI recently and has a court date in 2 weeks. He reports that he has tried on several occasions to quit alcohol on his own. However, he reports that when he stops drinking he feels "shaky, sweaty, anxious, and irritable" and thus resumes his alcohol intake. He also reports a history of having had a seizure after he abruptly discontinued his alcohol use during a few days more than 10 years ago.

Mr. Smith's last drink was about 8 hours prior to his arrival at the ED. The patient reports that during the last month, he has been feeling sad, had low energy levels, has difficulty falling and staying asleep, has ↓ appetite, and difficulty concentrating. He denies suicidal ideation but reports guilt over not being able to stop drinking. He denies a history of depression or anxiety, and has not received any psychiatric treatment in the past.

Upon presentation to ER the patient's breathalyzer was 0.110, he did not have symptoms of intoxication and his urine drug screen was negative. Vital signs were significant for blood pressure of 150/90 and pulse of 110 bpm. Complete blood count and electrolytes were within normal limits.

What is Mr. Smith's most likely diagnosis?

The patient described above has a diagnosis of alcohol dependence with physiological dependence. It is clear that the patient has exhibited symptoms of tolerance and withdrawal, has been using more alcohol than intended, and has made unsuccessful efforts to cut down. The patient also describes symptoms suggestive of a depressive disorder. The fact that his depressive symptoms began while abusing alcohol warrants a diagnosis of alcohol-induced depressive disorder. However, major depressive disorder should be ruled out once he remits his alcohol use. If his depressive symptoms are indeed substance-induced, they will improve and resolve with continuing sobriety.

What would be the next step in management?

Given the Mr. Smith's heavy chronic alcohol use and history of complicated withdrawal (ie, seizure), he should be admitted to an inpatient unit for close monitoring. Outpatient detoxification is not appropriate in this case. He will need to be medicated on a standing and PRN benzodiazepine (exact benzodiazepine sometimes varies depending on hospital's protocol), and monitored for signs of withdrawal.

Dependence

- The **CAGE questionnaire** is used to screen for alcohol abuse. Two or more "yes" answers are considered a positive screen:
  1. Have you ever wanted to **C**ut down on your drinking?
  2. Have you ever felt **A**nnoyed by criticism of your drinking?
  3. Have you ever felt **G**uilty about drinking?
  4. Have you ever taken a drink as an "**E**ye opener" (to prevent the shakes)?
- Biochemical markers are useful in detecting recent prolonged drinking; ongoing monitoring of biomarkers can help detect a relapse. Most commonly used biomarkers are BAL, liver function tests (LFTs—aspartate aminotransferase [AST], alanine aminotransferase [ALT]), gamma-glutamyl transpeptidase (GGT), carbohydrate-deficient transferrin (CDT), and mean corpuscular volume (MCV).

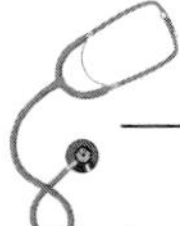

At-risk or heavy drinking for men is > 4 drinks per day or > 14 drinks per week. For women, it is > 3 drinks per day or > 7 drinks per week.

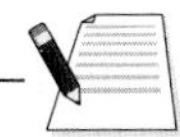

AST:ALT ratio ≥ 2:1 and elevated GGT suggest excessive alcohol use.

Medications for Alcohol Dependence

- Disulfiram (Antabuse):
  - Blocks the enzyme aldehyde dehydrogenase in the liver and causes aversive reaction to alcohol (flushing, headache, nausea/vomiting, palpitations, shortness of breath).
  - Contraindicated in severe cardiac disease, pregnancy, psychosis.

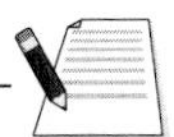

Alcohol can cause ↑ LFTs and macrocytosis (↑ MCV).

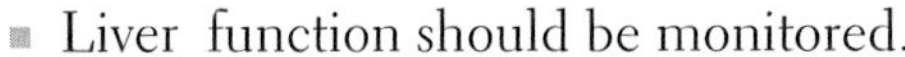

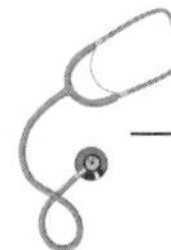

All patients with altered mental status should be given thiamine *before* glucose, or Wernicke-Korsakoff syndrome may be precipitated. Thiamine is a coenzyme used in carbohydrate metabolism.

- Liver function should be monitored.
- Best used in highly motivated patients, as medication adherence is an issue.
- Naltrexone (Revia, IM-Vivitrol):
  - Opioid receptor blocker.
  - Works by ↓ desire/craving and "high" associated with alcohol.
  - Greater benefit is seen in persons with family history of alcoholism.
  - In patients with physical opioid dependence, it will precipitate withdrawal.
- Acamprosate (Campral):
  - Structurally similar to GABA, thought to inhibit the glutamatergic system.
  - Should be started postdetoxification for relapse prevention in patients who have stopped drinking.
  - Major advantage is that it can be used in patients with liver disease.
  - Contraindicated in severe renal disease.
- Topiramate (Topamax):
  - Anticonvulsant that potentiates GABA and inhibits glutamate receptors.
  - Reduces cravings for alcohol.

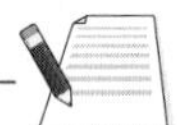

Delirium tremens is a dangerous form of alcohol withdrawal involving mental status and neurological changes. Symptoms include seizures (usually generalized tonic-clonic); visual and tactile hallucinations; and ↑ respiratory rate, heart rate, and blood pressure. Treatment includes anticonvulsants such as Dilantin (phenytoin) and sedatives such as benzodiazepines.

LONG-TERM COMPLICATIONS OF ALCOHOL INTAKE

- **Wernicke's encephalopathy:**
  - Caused by thiamine (vitamin B_1) deficiency resulting from poor nutrition.
  - Acute and can be reversed with thiamine therapy.
  - Features: Ataxia (broad-based), confusion, ocular abnormalities (nystagmus, gaze palsies).
- If left untreated, Wernicke's encephalopathy may progress to **Korsakoff syndrome:**
  - Chronic amnestic syndrome.
  - Reversible in only about 20% of patients.
  - Features: Impaired recent memory, anterograde amnesia, compensatory confabulation (unconsciously making up answers when memory has failed).

COCAINE

Cocaine blocks dopamine reuptake from the synaptic cleft, causing a stimulant effect. Dopamine plays a role in behavioral reinforcement ("reward" system of the brain).

Intoxication

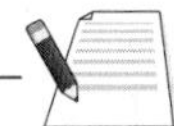

Cocaine overdose can cause death secondary to cardiac arrhythmia, MI, seizure, or respiratory depression.

- *General:* Euphoria, heightened self-esteem, ↑ or ↓ blood pressure, tachycardia or bradycardia, nausea, dilated pupils, weight loss, psychomotor agitation or depression, chills, and sweating.
- *Dangerous:* Respiratory depression, seizures, arrhythmias, paranoia, and hallucinations (especially tactile). Since cocaine is an indirect sympathomimetic, intoxication mimics the fight-or-flight response.
- *Deadly:* Cocaine's vasoconstrictive effect may result in myocardial infarction (MI) or stroke.

MANAGEMENT

- For mild-to-moderate agitation and anxiety: Reassurance of the patient and benzodiazepines.
- For severe agitation or psychosis: Antipsychotics (haloperidol).
- Symptomatic support (ie, control hypertension, arrhythmias).
- Temperature of > 102°F is a medical emergency and should be treated aggressively with ice bath, cooling blanket, and other supportive measures.

Dependence

Treatment of cocaine dependence includes:

- There is no FDA-approved pharmacotherapy for cocaine dependence.
- Off-label medications are sometimes used (disulfiram, aripiprazole).
- Psychological interventions (contingency management, group therapy, etc) are efficacious and are mainstay treatment.

Withdrawal

- Abrupt abstinence is **not** life threatening.
- Produces postintoxication depression ("crash"): Malaise, fatigue, hypersomnolence, depression, hunger, constricted pupils, vivid dreams, psychomotor agitation or retardation. Occasionally, these patients can become suicidal.
- With mild to moderate cocaine use, withdrawal symptoms resolve within 18 hours; with heavy, chronic use, they may last for weeks, but usually peak in several days.
- Treatment is supportive, but severe psychotic symptoms may warrant hospitalization.

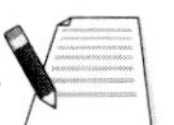

Heavy use may cause amphetamine psychosis, a psychotic state that may mimic schizophrenia.

AMPHETAMINES

- Classic amphetamines:
  - Block reuptake and facilitate release of dopamine and norepinephrine from nerve endings, causing a stimulant effect.
  - *Examples:* Dextroamphetamine (Dexedrine), methylphenidate (Ritalin), methamphetamine (Desoxyn, "ice," "speed," "crystal meth," "crank").
  - Methamphetamines are easily manufactured in home laboratories using over-the-counter medications (ie, pseudoephedrine).
  - They are used medically in the treatment of narcolepsy, attention deficit/hyperactivity disorder (ADHD), and depressive disorders.
- Substituted ("designer," "club drugs") amphetamines:
  - Release dopamine, norepinephrine, and serotonin from nerve endings.
  - *Examples*: MDMA ("ecstasy,") MDEA ("eve").
  - These substances are associated with dance clubs and raves.
  - Have both stimulant and hallucinogenic properties.
  - Serotonin syndrome is possible if designer amphetamines are combined with selective serotonin reuptake inhibitors (SSRIs).

Remember, the symptoms of amphetamine abuse are dilated pupils, ↑ libido, perspiration, respiratory depression, chest pain.

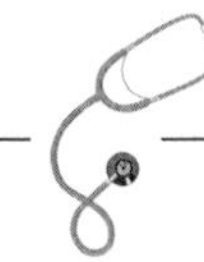

Chronic amphetamine use → acne and accelerated tooth decay ("meth mouth").

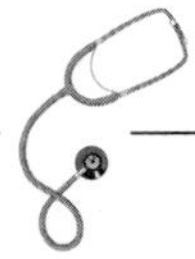

Amphetamine use is associated with ↑ tolerance, but also can → seizures.

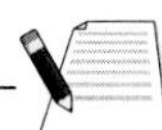

Ketamine ("special K") can produce tachycardia, tachypnea, hallucinations, and amnesia.

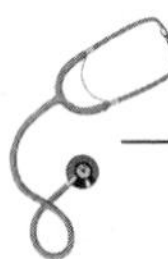

PCP intoxication symptoms—

RED DANES

Rage
Erythema (redness of skin)
Dilated pupils
Delusions
Amnesia
Nystagmus
Excitation
Skin dryness

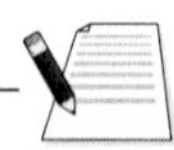

Rotatory nystagmus is pathognomonic for PCP intoxicaton.

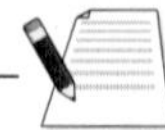

Tactile and visual hallucinations are found in both cocaine and PCP abuse.

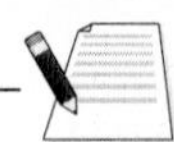

More than with other drugs, intoxication with PCP results in violence.

HIGH-YIELD FACTS

SUBSTANCE-RELATED DISORDERS

Intoxication

Clinical Presentation

- Amphetamine intoxication causes symptoms similar to those of cocaine (see above).
- MDMA and MDEA may induce sense of closeness to others.
- Overdose can → hyperthermia, dehydration (especially after a prolonged period of dancing in a club), and rhabdomyolysis → renal failure.
- Amphetamine withdrawal can → prolonged depression; occasionally, complications of their long half-life can cause psychosis.

Treatment

Rehydrate, correct electrolyte balance, and treat hyperthermia.

PHENCYCLIDINE (PCP)

PCP, or "angel dust," is a dissociative, hallucinogenic drug that antagonizes N-methyl-D-aspartate (NMDA) glutamate receptors and activates dopaminergic neurons. It can have stimulant or CNS depressant effects, depending on the dose taken.

- PCP can be smoked as "wet" (sprinkled on cigarette) or as a "joint" (sprinkled on marijuana).
- Ketamine is similar to PCP, but is less potent. Ketamine is sometimes used as a "date rape" drug, as it is odorless and tasteless.

Intoxication

Clinical Presentation

- Effects include agitation, depersonalization, hallucinations, synesthesia, impaired judgment, memory impairment, assaultiveness, **nystagmus** (rotary, horizontal, or vertical), ataxia, dysarthria, hypertension, tachycardia, muscle rigidity, and high tolerance to pain.
- Overdose can cause seizures, coma, and even death.

Treatment

- Monitor vitals, temperature, and electrolytes and minimize sensory stimulation.
- Use benzodiazepines (lorazepam) to treat agitation, anxiety, muscle spasms, and seizures.
- Use antipsychotics (haloperidol) to control severe agitation or psychotic symptoms.

Withdrawal

No withdrawal syndrome, but "flashbacks" (recurrence of intoxication symptoms due to release of the drug from body lipid stores) may occur.

SEDATIVES-HYPNOTICS

Agents in the sedatives-hypnotics category include benzodiazepines, barbiturates, zolpidem, zaleplon, gamma-hydroxybutyrate (GHB), meprobamate, and others. These medications, especially benzodiazepines, are highly abused in the United States, as they are more readily available than other drugs such as cocaine or opioids.

- Benzodiazepines (BDZs):
  - Commonly used in the treatment of anxiety disorders.
  - Easily obtained via prescription from physician offices and emergency departments.
  - Potentiate the effects of GABA by ↑ the frequency of chloride channel opening.
- Barbiturates:
  - Used in the treatment of epilepsy and as anesthetics.
  - Potentiate the effects of GABA by ↑ the duration of chloride channel opening.
  - At high doses, barbiturates act as direct GABA agonists and have a lower margin of safety relative to BDZs.
  - They are synergistic in combination BDZs and barbiturates (as well as other CNS depressants); respiratory depression can occur as a complication.

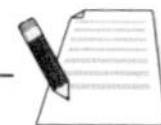

Gamma-hydroxybutyrate (GHB) is a dose-specific CNS depressant that produces memory loss, respiratory distress, and coma. It is commonly used as a date-rape drug.

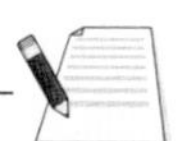

Barbiturate withdrawal can be **deadly.** Of all the kinds of drug withdrawals, withdrawal from barbiturates has the highest mortality rate. Although barbiturate abuse is still a major problem, abuse of other depressants, such as benzodiazepines, is becoming more common.

Intoxication

Clinical Presentation

- Intoxication with sedatives produces drowsiness, confusion, hypotension, slurred speech, incoordination, ataxia, mood lability, impaired judgment, nystagmus, respiratory depression, and coma or death in overdose.
- Symptoms are synergistic when combined with EtOH or opioids/narcotics.
- Long-term sedative use may → dependence and may cause depressive symptoms.

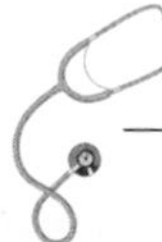

Flumazenil is a very short-acting BDZ antagonist used for treating BDZ overdose. Use with caution when treating overdose, as it may precipitate seizures.

Treatment

- Maintain airway, breathing, and circulation. Monitor vital signs.
- Activated charcoal and gastric lavage to prevent further gastrointestinal absorption (if drug was ingested in the prior 4–6 hours).
- For *barbiturates only:* Alkalinize urine with sodium bicarbonate to promote renal excretion.
- For *benzodiazepines only:* Flumazenil in overdose.
- Supportive care—improve respiratory status, control hypotension.

Naloxone is the treatment of choice for opiate overdose.

Withdrawal

Abrupt abstinence after chronic use can be ***life threatening.*** While physiological dependence is more likely with short-acting agents, longer-acting agents can also cause dependence and withdrawal symptoms.

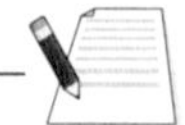

In general, withdrawal from drugs that are sedating is life threatening, while withdrawal from stimulants is not.

Clinical Presentation

Signs and symptoms of withdrawal are the same as these of EtOH withdrawal. Tonic-clonic seizures may occur and can be life threatening.

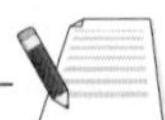

The opioid dextromethorphan is a common ingredient in cough syrup.

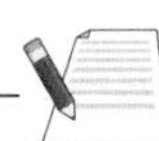

Infection secondary to needle sharing is the most common cause of death from street heroin usage.

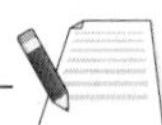

Opiate intoxication: nausea, vomiting, sedation, ↓ pain perception, ↓ gastrointestinal motility, pupil constriction. Also respiratory depression, which *can* kill you.

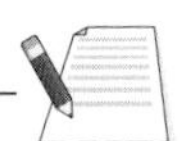

Meperidine is the exception to opioids producing miosis. "**De**merol **Di**lates pupils."

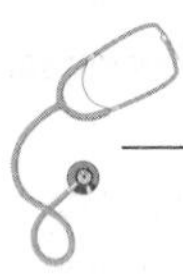

Classic triad of opioid overdose—

Rebels Admire Morphine

Respiratory depression
Altered mental status
Miosis

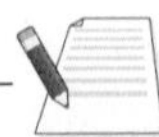

Eating poppy seed bagels or muffins can result in a urine drug screen that is positive for opioids.

Treatment

- Benzodiazepine taper.
- Carbamazepine or valproic acid taper may be used for seizure prevention.

OPIOIDS

- Opioid medications and drugs of abuse stimulate opiate receptors (mu, kappa, and delta), which are normally stimulated by endogenous opiates and are involved in analgesia, sedation, and dependence. Examples include heroin, oxycodone, codeine, dextromethorphan, morphine, methadone, and meperidine (Demerol).
- Opioids also have effects on the dopaminergic system, which mediates their addictive and rewarding properties.
- Prescription opioids (OxyContin [oxycodone], Vicodin [hydrocodone/acetaminophen], and Percocet [oxycodone/acetaminophen]), not heroin, are most commonly abused.
- Behaviors such as losing medication, "doctor shopping," and running out of medication early should alert clinician of possible misuse.

Intoxication

Clinical Presentation

- Opioid intoxication causes drowsiness, nausea/vomiting, constipation, slurred speech, **constricted pupils**, seizures, and respiratory depression, which may progress to coma or death in overdose.
- Meperidine and monoamine oxidase inhibitors taken in combination may cause the **serotonin syndrome:** hyperthermia, confusion, hyper- or hypotension, and muscular rigidity.

Treatment

- Ensure adequate airway, breathing, and circulation.
- In overdose, administration of naloxone or naltrexone (opioid antagonists) will improve respiratory depression but may cause severe withdrawal in an opioid-dependent patient.
- Ventilatory support may be required.

Dependence

See Table 6-4 for treatment of opioid dependence.

Withdrawal

- While not life threatening, abstinence in the opioid-dependent individual → an unpleasant withdrawal syndrome characterized by dysphoria, insomnia, lacrimation, rhinorrhea, yawning, weakness, sweating, piloerection, nausea/vomiting, fever, dilated pupils, abdominal cramps, arthralgia, myalgia, hypertension, tachycardia, craving.
- Treatment includes:
  - Moderate symptoms: Symptomatic treatment with clonidine (for autonomic signs and symptoms of withdrawal), nonsteroidal anti-

TABLE 6-4. Pharmacological Treatment of Opioid Dependence

MEDICATION	MECHANISM	PROS	CONS
Methadone	Long-acting opioid receptor agonist	Administered once daily. Significantly reduces morbidity and mortality in opioid-dependent persons. "Gold standard" treatment in pregnant opioid-dependent women.	Restricted to federally licensed substance abuse treatment programs. Can cause QTc interval prolongation; thus, screening electrocardiogram is indicated for certain patients such as those with cardiac disease.
Buprenorphine	Partial opioid receptor agonist	Sublingual preparation that is safer than methadone, as its effects reach a plateau and make overdose unlikely. Comes as Suboxone, which contains buprenorphine and naloxone; more commonly used, as this preparation limits diversion.	Available by prescription from office-based physicians.
Naltrexone	Competitive opioid antagonist, precipitates withdrawal if used within 7 days of heroin use	It is a good choice for highly motivated patients such as health care professionals.	Compliance is an issue.

inflammatory drugs (NSAIDs) for pain, dicyclomine for abdominal cramps, etc.
- Severe symptoms: Detox with buprenorphine or methadone.
- Monitor degree of withdrawal with COWS (Clinical Opioid Withdrawal Scale), which uses objective measures (ie, pulse, pupil size, tremor) to assess withdrawal severity.

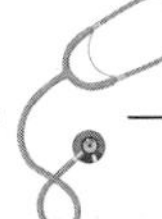

Rapid recovery of consciousness following the administration of intravenous (IV) naloxone (opioid antagonist) is consistent with opioid overdose.

HALLUCINOGENS

Hallucinogenic drugs of abuse include psilocybin (mushrooms), mescaline (peyote cactus), and lysergic acid diethylamide (LSD). Pharmacological effects vary, but LSD is believed to act on the serotonergic system. Hallucinogens do not cause physical dependence or withdrawal, though users can rarely develop psychological dependence.

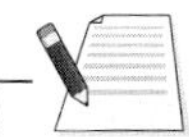

Remember the withdrawal symptoms of opiates: anxiety, insomnia, anorexia, fever, rhinorrhea, piloerection. This *not* life threatening.

Intoxication

- Effects include perceptual changes (illusions, hallucinations, body image distortions, synesthesia), labile affect, dilated pupils, tachycardia, hypertension, hyperthermia, tremors, incoordination, sweating, and palpitations.
- Usually lasts 6–12 hours, but may last for several days.

- May have a "bad trip" that consists of marked anxiety, panic, and psychotic symptoms (paranoia, hallucinations).
- **Treatment:** Monitor for dangerous behavior and reassure patient. Use benzodiazepines or antipsychotics if necessary for agitated psychosis.

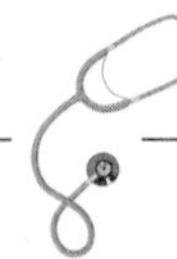

Withdrawal from opioids is *not* life threatening, but it does cause severe symptoms

Withdrawal

No withdrawal syndrome is produced, but with long-term LSD use, patients may experience "flashbacks" later in life.

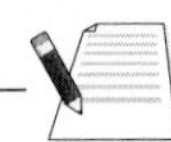

An LSD flashback is a recurrence of symptoms mimicking prior LSD trip that occurs spontaneously and lasts for minutes to hours.

MARIJUANA

- Cannabis ("marijuana," "pot," "weed," "grass") is the world's most commonly used illicit substance.
- The main active component in cannabis is THC (tetrahydrocannabinol).
- Cannabinoid receptors in the brain inhibit adenylate cyclase.
- Marijuana has been shown to successfully treat nausea in chemotherapy patients, ↑ appetite in AIDS patients, and ↓ intraocular pressure, muscle spasms, and tremor.

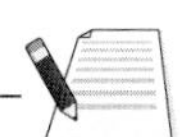

Dronabinol is a pill form of THC that is FDA-approved for certain indications.

Intoxication

- Marijuana causes euphoria, anxiety, impaired motor coordination, perceptual disturbances (sensation of slowed time), mild tachycardia, anxiety, **conjunctival injection (red eyes)**, dry mouth, and ↑ appetite ("the munchies").
- Cannabis-induced psychotic disorders with paranoia, hallucinations, and/or delusions may occur. There is no overdose syndrome of marijuana use.
- Marijuana dependence occurs in approximately 5% of users.
- Chronic use may cause respiratory problems such as asthma and chronic bronchitis, suppression of immune system, and possible effects on reproductive hormones.
- **Treatment:** Supportive, psychosocial interventions (eg, contingency management, groups, etc).

Withdrawal

- Withdrawal symptoms may include irritability, anxiety, restlessness, aggression, strange dreams, depression, headaches, sweating, insomnia, nausea, craving, and ↓ appetite.
- **Treatment:** Supportive and symptomatic.

INHALANTS

- Inhalants include a broad range of drugs that are inhaled and absorbed through the lungs.
- Inhalants generally act as CNS depressants.

- User is typically a preadolescent or adolescent; rate of use is similar between boys and girls.
- *Examples:* Solvents, glue, paint thinners, fuels, isobutyl nitrates ("huff," "laughing gas," "rush," "bolt").

Intoxication

- **Effects:** Perceptual disturbances, psychosis (especially paranoid states), lethargy, dizziness, nausea/vomiting, headache, nystagmus, tremor, muscle weakness, hyporeflexia, ataxia, slurred speech, euphoria, hypoxia, clouding of consciousness, stupor, or coma.
- Acute intoxication lasts minutes. A stupor may last for hours.
- **Overdose:** May be fatal secondary to respiratory depression or cardiac arrhythmias.
- Long-term use may cause permanent damage to CNS (eg, dementia, impaired memory, epilepsy, reduced IQ), peripheral nervous system (PNS), liver, kidney, heart, and muscle.
- **Treatment:** Monitor airway, breathing, and circulation.
- Identify solvent because some (ie, leaded gasoline) may require chelation.

Withdrawal

A withdrawal syndrome does not usually occur, but symptoms may include irritability, sleep disturbance, nausea, vomiting, diaphoresis, tachycardia, and occasionally hallucinations and delusions.

CAFFEINE

Caffeine is the most commonly used psychoactive substance in the United States, usually in the form of coffee or tea. It acts as an adenosine antagonist, causing ↑ cyclic adenosine monophosphate (cAMP) and a stimulant effect via the dopaminergic system.

Overdose

- 250 mg (2–3 cups of coffee): Anxiety, insomnia, muscle twitching, rambling speech, flushed face, diuresis, gastrointestinal disturbance, restlessness, excitement, and tachycardia.
- > 1 g: May cause tinnitus, severe agitation, visual light flashes, and cardiac arrhythmias.
- >10 g: Death may occur secondary to seizures and respiratory failure.
- **Treatment:** Supportive and symptomatic.

Withdrawal

- Caffeine withdrawal symptoms occur in 50–75% of caffeine users if cessation is abrupt.
- Withdrawal symptoms include headache, fatigue, irritability, nausea, vomiting, drowsiness, anxiety, muscle pain, and mild depression.
- Usually resolve within 1 week.

NICOTINE

- Nicotine is derived from the tobacco plant, and stimulates nicotinic receptors in autonomic ganglia of the sympathetic and parasympathetic nervous systems. It is highly addictive through its effects on the dopaminergic system.
- Smoking → tolerance and physical dependence (ie, prominent craving).
- Cigarette smoking is the leading cause of preventable morbidity and mortality in the United States, posing many health risks including chronic obstructive pulmonary disease (COPD) and various cancers.
- Current smoking prevalence is about 21% of U.S. adults.
- **Effects:** Restlessness, insomnia, anxiety, and ↑ gastrointestinal motility.
- **Withdrawal symptoms:** Intense craving, dysphoria, anxiety, poor concentration, ↓ heart rate, ↑ appetite, irritability, restlessness, and insomnia.

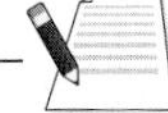

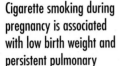

Cigarette smoking during pregnancy is associated with low birth weight and persistent pulmonary hypertension of the newborn.

Treatment of Nicotine Dependence

FDA-approved pharmacotherapy:

- Varenicline (Chantix): $\alpha 4\beta 2$ nicotinic cholinergic receptor (nAChR) partial agonist that mimics the action of nicotine and prevents withdrawal symptoms.
- Bupropion (Zyban): Antidepressant that is also a partial agonist at nAChR and inhibitor of dopamine reuptake; helps reduce withdrawal symptoms.
- Nicotine replacement therapy (NRT): Available as transdermal patch, gum, lozenge, nasal spray, and inhaler.
- Behavioral counseling should be part of every treatment.
- Relapse after abstinence is common.

HIGH-YIELD FACTS IN

Cognitive Disorders

DEFINITION

A cognitive disorder is a significant change in cognition from a previous level of functioning. It may affect memory, attention, language, and judgment. Cognitive disorders may be associated with abnormalities of the central nervous system, a general medical condition, medications, or substance use. The two main types of cognitive disorders are delirium and dementia (see Table 7-4).

Mrs. Brown is an 83-year-old woman who was admitted to the general medical hospital after presenting with fever and altered mental status. The patient's home aide nurse, reports that she was in her usual state of health until the day prior to her admission, when she was observed to be confused and talking to her mother, who had been deceased for years. Reportedly, mental status improved to near baseline a few hours later. However, the nurse aide later called the ambulance to bring the patient into the hospital because she was observed calling 911, stating that people were in her house trying to kill her. On examination, Mrs. Brown is somnolent, has difficulty concentrating during the interview, and requires questions to be repeated frequently. She is restless, paranoid, disoriented to place and time, and is noted to be addressing the chair in the room as her mother. She also appears to be gesturing and calling her dog to come and sit next to her.

In speaking with patient's family, you learn that Mrs. Brown has had progressive memory deficits. Family members report that she initially confused her grandchildren's names and had difficulty remembering recent conversations with them. As the years passed, they reported that her symptoms worsened, and they described an episode during which she forgot to turn off the stove and almost burned her house down. Because of this, Mrs. Brown has had a 24-hour home health aide for the past 2 years. She is no longer able to manage her finances or drive and needs assistance when performing her activities of daily living.

What is her most likely diagnosis?

Mrs. Brown's most likely diagnosis is delirium. She presents with a sudden change in cognition as manifested by confusion, disorientation, paranoia, and hallucinations. She shows a disturbance of consciousness with reduced ability to focus, sustain, or shift attention. This is evidenced by her somnolence, poor concentration, and the need to have questions repeated. Mrs. Brown also shows the development of disorientation to place and time and appears to be responding to perceptual disturbances. Finally, she has had an acute change from her baseline behavior, and her symptoms waxed and waned throughout the day, representing the typical fluctuation of symptoms found in delirium. Mrs. Brown presented with fever, likely secondary to an infection, which is the most likely cause of her symptoms. If this is confirmed, her diagnosis is then stated as delirium due to a general medical condition.

Collateral information obtained from family members points to a prior diagnosis of dementia. Mrs. Brown has a history of memory impairment that began gradually and has progressively declined. There is also history of impairment in executive functioning, and she is no longer able to care for herself. Remember that dementia is a risk factor for the development of delirium.

How can the paranoia and agitation be best treated?

While not part of diagnostic criteria, psychomotor symptoms often accompany delirium and can show either psychomotor agitation or retardation. Agitation can → injury to the patient and/or staff members. Psychotropic medications, particularly antipsychotics, can be used for symptomatic treatment of delirium while etiologic causes are treated. Low-dose haloperidol is commonly used in this situation and has the advantage of being able to be given orally, intramuscularly, or intravenously. Benzodiazepines are often given for agitation, but many worsen delirium and should be reserved for delirium as a result of alcohol or benzodiazepine withdrawal.

Delirium is common in intensive care unit setting/acute medical illness and has ↑ incidence in children and elderly.

DELIRIUM

You are consulted on a 57-year-old man who presents with tremor, extrapyramidal symptoms, frontal dizziness, and sluggish pupillary reflexes. *What is the likely diagnosis?* Tertiary syphilis. *Next step:* Order Venereal Disease Research Laboratory test (VDRL). VDRL and thyroid-stimulating hormone (TSH) are part of every initial psychiatric workup.

- Delirium is a waxing-and-waning change in a patient's level of consciousness. It is very common and has many different presentations, causing it to be underrecognized and underdiagnosed.
- It can be caused by virtually any medical disorder, and it has a high morbidity and mortality if untreated.
- It can last from days to weeks, and may become chronic.
- It can also be referred to by the terms *encephalopathy, acute organic brain syndrome, acute confusional state, acute toxic psychosis,* and *ICU psychosis.*

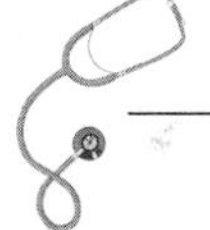

Causes of delirium—AEIOU TIPS

Alcohol/drugs toxicity or withdrawal
Electrolyte abnormality
Iatrogenic (anticholinergics, benzodiazepines, antiepileptics, blood pressure medicines, insulin, hypoglycemics, narcotics, steroids, H_2 receptor blockers, NSAIDs, antibiotics, antiparkinsonians)
Oxygen hypoxia (bleeding, central venous, pulmonary)
Uremia/hepatic encephalopathy
Trauma
Infection
Poisons
Seizures (postictal), **S**troke

EPIDEMIOLOGY

- Ten to thirty percent of medically admitted patients exhibit delirium.
- Common in elderly patients, intensive care unit (ICU) patients, postop surgery patients, and cancer patients.

RISK FACTORS

- Advanced age
- Preexisting brain damage (dementia, cerebrovascular accident [CVA], tumor)
- Prior history of delirium
- Alcohol dependence
- Diabetes
- Cancer
- Sensory impairment or blindness
- Malnutrition
- Male gender

ETIOLOGY

- Almost any medical condition can cause delirium. See Table 7-1 for clinical scenarios of delirium.
- Infection, medications, substance intoxication or withdrawal, and electrolyte imbalances are the most common causes.

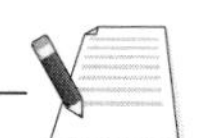

Visual hallucinations and short attention span are two typical symptoms of delirium.

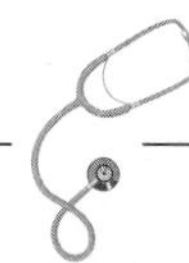

Impairment in recent memory is most common finding in delirium.

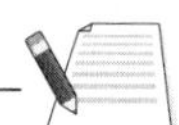

The hallmark of delirium is waxing and waning of symptoms. Patient will have changes in their mental status over time and may have "lucid intervals."

CLINICAL MANIFESTATIONS

- Disorientation: Usually to time or place, rarely to person.
- Language disturbances: Dysarthria, dysnomia, dysgraphia, and aphasia.
- Changes in speech: Slow, pressured, rambling, or disorganized.
- Perceptual disturbances: Misinterpretations, illusions, or hallucinations.
- Sleep disturbances: Sundowning with daytime drowsiness and nighttime insomnia and confusion.
- Disturbed psychomotor behavior: Hyperactivity or hypoactivity, may shift from one extreme to the other over the course of a day.
- Emotional disturbances: Anxiety, fear, depression, irritability, anger, apathy, euphoria (may mimic other psychiatric conditions).
- Perseveration: Inability to shift attention appropriately, making conversations difficult.

DIAGNOSIS

Diagnostic and Statistical Manual of Mental Disorders, 4th edition, Text Revision (DSM-IV-TR) criteria:

1. Disturbance of consciousness (ie, reduced clarity of awareness of the environment) with reduced ability to focus, sustain, or shift attention.
2. A change in cognition (such as memory deficit, disorientation, language disturbance) or the development of a perceptual disturbance that is not better accounted for by a preexisting, established, or evolving dementia.
3. The disturbance develops over a short period of time (usually hours to days) and tends to fluctuate during the course of the day.

TABLE 7-1. Clinical Scenarios of Delirium on the Exam

SCENARIO	THINK	CONFIRMATORY DIAGNOSTIC TESTS
Delirium + hemiparesis or other focal neurological signs and symptoms	CVA or mass lesion	Brain CT/MRI
Delirium + elevated blood pressure + papilledema	Hypertensive encephalopathy	Brain CT/MRI
Delirium + dilated pupils + tachycardia	Drug intoxication	Urine toxicology screen
Delirium + fever + nuchal rigidity + photophobia	Meningitis	Lumbar puncture
Delirium + tachycardia + tremor + thyromegaly	Thyrotoxicosis	T_4, TSH

CVA, cerebrovascular accident; CT, computed tomography; MRI, magnetic resonance imaging; T_4, thyroxine; TSH, thyroid-stimulating hormone.

TREATMENT

- Rule out life-threatening causes.
- Definitive treatment requires the identification and treatment of the underlying conditions; for example, hypothyroidism, electrolyte imbalances, urinary tract infection.
- Supportive care: Maintain hydration and nutrition.
- Patient safety:
  - One-on-one nursing observation.
  - Frequently orient patient.
  - Avoid napping and keep lights on or shades open during the day to correct sleep cycle.
- Psychotropic medications can be used for symptomatic treatment of delirium, particularly agitation:
  - Antipsychotics first line: Haloperidol is most studied and can be given PO/IM/IV.
  - Benzodiazepines are usually avoided unless delirium is secondary to alcohol or benzodiazepine withdrawal.
  - Benzodiazepines can cause/prolong delirium.

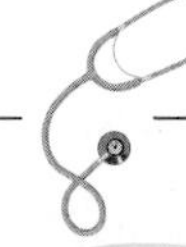

Avoid using benzodiazepines in delirious patients, as they will often exacerbate the delirium.

DEMENTIA

- Dementia is an impairment of memory and other cognitive functions (language skills, behavior, and personality) without alteration in the level of consciousness.
- Dementia is a major cause of disability in the elderly.
- Most forms of dementia are progressive and irreversible.
- Dementia may be etiologically related to a general medical condition, the persisting effects of substance use, or a combination of these factors. See Table 7-2 for clinical scenarios of dementia.
- Prevalence almost doubles every 5 years (1.5% at 60 years, 40% at 90 years).
- There is a similar pattern of dementia subtypes across the world.
- Most common: Alzheimer's (50–70%).
- Second most common: Vascular dementia (15–25%).

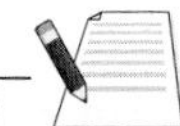

If a patient presents with dementia but has a normal computed tomographic (CT) scan, a complete metabolic panel and magnetic resonance imaging (MRI) should be ordered.

DIFFERENTIAL DIAGNOSIS

- Psychiatric: Depression, delirium, malingering.
- Structural: Benign forgetfulness of normal aging, Parkinson's disease, Huntington disease, Down syndrome, head trauma, brain tumor, normal pressure hydrocephalus, multiple sclerosis, subdural hematoma.
- Metabolic: Hypothyroidism, hypoxia, malnutrition (B_{12}, folate, or thiamine deficiency), Wilson disease, lead toxicity.
- Infectious: Lyme disease, HIV dementia, Creutzfeldt-Jakob disease, neurosyphilis, meningitis, encephalitis.
- Drugs: Alcohol (chronic and acute), anticholinergics, sedatives.

DIAGNOSIS

DSM-IV-TR criteria:

1. The development of multiple cognitive deficits manifested by both:
   - Memory impairment (impaired ability to learn new information or to recall previously learned information)

TABLE 7-2. Clinical Scenarios of Dementia on the Exam

Scenario	Think	Confirmatory/ Diagnostic Tests
Dementia with stepwise ↑ in severity + focal neurological signs	Multi-infarct dementia	CT/MRI
Dementia + cogwheel rigidity + resting tremor	Lewy body dementia Parkinson disease	Clinical
Dementia + gait apraxia + urinary incontinence + dilated cerebral ventricles	Normal pressure hydrocephalus	CT/MRI
Dementia + obesity + coarse hair + constipation + cold intolerance	Hypothyroidism	T_4, TSH
Dementia + diminished position and vibration sensation + megaloblasts on CBC	Vitamin B_{12} deficiency	Serum B_{12}
Dementia + tremor + abnormal LFTs + Kayser–Fleischer rings	Wilson disease	Ceruloplasmin
Dementia + diminished position and vibration sensation + **A**rgyll **R**obertson **P**upils (**A**ccommodation **R**esponse **P**resent, response to light absent)	Neurosyphilis	CSF FTA-ABS or CSF VDRL

CBC, complete blood count; CSF, cerebrospinal fluid; CT, computed tomography; FTA-ABS, fluorescent treponemal antibody absorption test; LFT, liver function test; MRI, magnetic resonance imaging; T_4, thyroxine; TSH, thyroid-stimulating hormone; VDRL, Venereal Disease Research Laboratory.

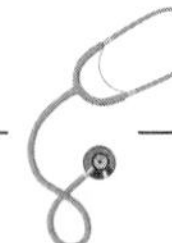

Workup for reversible causes of dementia:

- CBC
- Electrolytes
- TFTs
- VDRL/RPR
- B_{12} and folate levels
- Brain CT or MRI

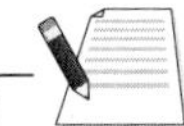

Hypothyroidism can cause *reversible* dementia. It is typically accompanied by depressed mood and lethargy.

- One (or more) of the following cognitive disturbances:
  - Aphasia (language disturbance)
  - Apraxia (impaired ability to carry out motor activities despite intact motor function)
  - Agnosia (failure to recognize or identify objects despite intact sensory function)
  - Disturbance in executive functioning (ie, planning, organizing, sequencing, abstracting)

2. The cognitive deficits in criteria A1 and A2 each cause significant impairment in social or occupational functioning and represent a significant decline from a previous level of functioning.
3. The deficits do not occur exclusively during the course of a delirium.

Associated features include:

- Delusions and hallucinations occur in approximately 30% of demented patients.
- Affective symptoms, including depression and anxiety, are seen in 40–50% of patients.
- Personality changes are also common.

The **Mini Mental State Exam (MMSE)** is a screening test used commonly due to its speed and ease of administration (see Table 7-3).

- Assesses orientation to time and place, attention/concentration, language, constructional ability, and immediate and delayed recall.

TABLE 7-3. Performing the Mini-Mental State Exam

1. Orientation	
What is the date, month, year?	5 points
Where are we (state, city, hospital)?	5 points
2. Registration	
Name three objects and repeat them.	3 points
3. Attention and calculation	
Serial 7s (subtract 7 from 100 and continue subtracting 7 from each answer) or spell "world" backward.	5 points
4. Recall	
Name the three objects above 5 minutes later.	3 points
5. Language	
Name a pen and a clock.	2 points
Say, "No ifs, ands, or buts."	1 points
Three-step command: Take a pencil in your right hand, put in your left hand, then put it on the floor.	3 points
6. Read and obey the following:	
Close your eyes.	1 point
Write a sentence.	1 point
Copy design.	1 point
TOTAL	**30 points**

- Sensitive for dementia, particularly moderate to severe forms.
- Lacks specificity; low scores may signal important changes in cognition.
- Presence and nature of cognitive impairment should not be diagnosed on the basis of MMSE scores alone.
- Norm tables are available to adjust for age and education:
  - Perfect score: 30
  - Dysfunction: < 25

Alzheimer Disease

- Alzheimer disease is the most common type of dementia and affects approximately 4.5 million in the United States.

TABLE 7-4. Delirium Versus Dementia

Delirium	Dementia
Clouding of consciousness	Loss of memory/intellectual ability
Acute onset	Insidious onset
Lasts 3 days to 2 weeks	Lasts months to years
Orientation impaired	Orientation often impaired
Immediate/recent memory impaired	Recent and remote memory impaired
Visual hallucinations common	Hallucinations less common
Symptoms fluctuate, often worse at night	Symptoms stable throughout day
Usually reversible	15% reversible
Awareness reduced	Awareness clear
Electroencephalographic (EEG) changes (fast waves or generalized slowing)	No EEG changes

- It affects women three times more than men, and its presence in one first-degree relative ↑ the risk fourfold.
- These patients have a ↓ in acetylcholine due to a loss of noradrenergic neurons in the basal ceruleus and ↓ choline acetyltransferase (required for acetylcholine synthesis).

Clinical Manifestations

- Gradual progressive decline in cognitive functions, especially memory and language.
- Personality changes, mood swings, and paranoia are very common.
- Motor and sensory symptoms are absent until late in the course of the illness.
- Gradual and progressive course, typically 10 years from diagnosis to death.

Diagnosis

- Remains a clinical diagnosis.
- Neuropsychological testing is helpful.
- Before death, it is a diagnosis of exclusion (definitive diagnosis is possible only at postmortem).
- **Genetics:**
  - Alzheimer genes (presenelin I, presenelin II, amyloid precursor protein (APP):
    - Genes are rare accounting for only 5% of cases, usually early onset.
    - Most cases, especially after 65, are sporadic.
  - Major susceptibility gene is apolipoprotein e4 (*APOe4*):
    - Homozygous (2% of population): 50–90% chance of developing dementia by age 85.

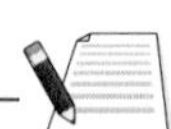

Senile plaques and neurofibrillary tangles are not unique to Alzheimer—they are also found in Down syndrome and normal aging.

- Heterozygous (15% of population): 45% chance of developing dementia by age 85
- Twenty percent chance in general population.
- Amyloid cascade hypothesis is the dominant explanation for Alzheimer disease:
  - Excess of Aβ peptides either by overproduction or diminished clearance.
  - APP, presenelin I, and presenelin II patients are lifelong overproducers.
  - Sporadic cases result from failure of metabolism and degradation.
- Postmortem findings:
  - Gross: Diffuse atrophy with enlarge ventricles and flattened sulci.
  - Microscopic: Senile plaques and neurofibrillary tangles.
  - Neuritic plaques, but not neufibrillary tangles, correlate with severity of dementia.

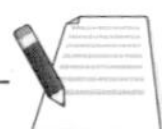

Pathological examination of the brain (at autopsy) is the only way to definitively diagnose Alzheimer disease.

Adults with Down sydrome are at ↑ risk of developing Alzheimer disease.

TREATMENT

- No cure or truly effective treatment.
- Physical and emotional support, proper nutrition, exercise, and supervision.
- Cholinesterace inhibitors:
  - Approved for mild-to-moderate disease
  - Able to slow cognitive decline for 6–12 months
  - *Examples:* Tacrine (Cognex), donepezil (Aricept), rivastigmine (Exelon), galantamine (Razadyne)
- NMDA antagonists:
  - Approved for moderate-to-severe disease
  - *Example:* Memantine (Namenda)

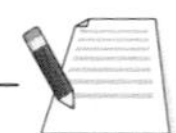

The presence of multiple infarcts on imaging does not automatically imply vascular dementia.

A patient with vascular dementia typically has chronically progressing dementia with multiple small lacunar infarcts (small vessel disease) on CT.

Vascular Dementia

A 68-year-old woman presents with crying at the slightest provocation and some slight confusion. This is new behavior, according to her daughter. Her history is significant for hypertension and transient ischemic attacks (TIAs). Exam reveals a carotid bruit. *What is the likely diagnosis?* Cerebrovascular accident (CVA).

A stroke to the frontal lobe can → symptoms of schizophrenia, bipolar I disorder, and depression.

Vascular dementia is the second most common form of dementia. It is caused by microvascular disease in the brain that produces multiple small infarcts. A substantial infarct burden must accumulate before dementia develops.

RISK FACTORS

- Stroke
- Diabetes mellitus
- Hypertension
- APOe4
- Two times more likely in men than in women

Clinical Manifestations

- May follow a single strategic infarct, multiple cortical or lacunar infarcts, or a microvascular insult.
- Step-wise deterioration.
- No specific pattern of cognitive deficits defines vascular dementia.
- Neuropsychological testing may not differentiate vascular dementia from Alzheimer disease.
- Lateralizing signs: Spasticity, hemiparesis, ataxia, pseudobalbar palsy (extreme emotional lability, abnormal speech cadence, dysphagia, abnormal reflexes).
- Depression, anger, and paranoia are common.

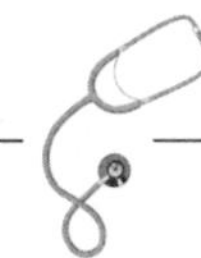

Classically, patients with vascular dementia have a **stepwise loss of function** as the microinfarcts add up.

Treatment

- No cure or truly effective treatment.
- Physical and emotional support, proper nutrition, exercise, and supervision.
- Cholinesterase inhibitors have been used successfully in patient with vascular dementia.
- Antihypertensive therapy may prevent onset of vascular dementia.
- Treatment of symptoms as necessary.

Lewy Body Dementia (LBD)

Lewy body dementia is the third most common dementia (accounting for 10–15%). It is caused by Lewy bodies and Lewy neurites (pathologic aggregations of alpha-synuclein) in the brain, primarily in the basal ganglia.

Clinical Manifestations

- Progressive cognitive decline.
- Waxing and waning of cognition is core feature.
- Visual hallucinations—usually vivid, colorful, and well-formed images of animals or people.
- Paranoid delusions are common.
- Parkinsonism (without exposure to neuroleptics) is core feature (tremor, bradykinesia, rigidity, shuffling gait, masked facies, stooped posture, retropulsion).
- Sensitivity to neuroleptics.
- Rapid eye movement (REM) sleep behavior disorder is common.

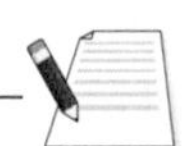

Core features of Lewy body dementia are waxing and waning, parkinsonism, visual hallucinations, and sensitivity to neuroleptics.

Diagnosis

- Strong similarities to Parkinson disease dementia:
  - Onset of dementia within 12 months of parkinsonism symptoms.
  - Dementia that begins more than 12 months after the parkinsonism symptoms is classified as Parkinson disease dementia.
- Lewy neurites are more closely linked with clinical symptoms than are Lewy bodies.

Treatment

- Cholinesterase inhibitors help improve visual hallucinations.
- Psychostimulants, levodopa/carbidopa, and dopamine agonists may improve cognition, apathy, and psychomotor slowing.

- Atypical neuroleptics have been slightly effective in stopping delusions and agitation.
- Clonazepam (Klonopin) treatment for REM sleep behavior disorder.

Pick Disease/Frontotemporal Dementia (FTD)

- FTD includes a diverse group of clinical and pathological disorders that typically present between the ages of 45 and 65.
- Approximately 20–30% are familial and may be associated with mutation in the progranulin or *MAPT* gene.
- The mean duration of illness to death is 4–6 years.

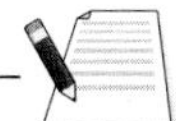

Pick disease → a more rapid progression to death than Alzheimer dementia.

Clinical Manifestations

- Profound changes in personality and social conduct.
- Usually present at the initial presentation of the patient.
- Disinhibited verbal, physical, and sexual behavior.
- Echolalia, overeating, oral exploration of inanimate objects.
- Lack emotional warmth, empathy or sympathy.
- Poor insight about behavioral alterations.
- Cognitive deficits in attention, abstraction, planning, and problem solving.
- Memory, language, and spatial functions are well preserved.

Pathology

- Marked atrophy of the frontal and temporal lobes
- Neuronal loss, microvacuolization, and astrocytic gliosis in cortical layer II
- Only moderate correlation between clinical and pathological findings

Treatment

Anticholinergic medications and antidepressants have consistently shown to improve behavioral symptoms but not cognition.

HIV-Associated Dementia (HAD)

HAD is the most common dementia caused by infectious disease, and its prevalence is increasing as patients live longer with illness. It is caused by infections due to neutropenia, as well as direct effects of the virus on cells.

Risk Factors

- Duration of illness
- Low CD4
- High viral loads

Clinical Manifestations

- Rapid decline in cognition, behavior, motor ability
- Poor memory and impaired concentration
- Psychomotor retardation
- Apathy and social withdrawal
- Depression
- Language usually preserved

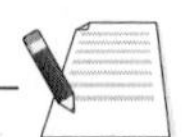

A ↓ in viral load is often accompanied by an improvement in AIDS-related dementia.

TREATMENT

- Highly active antiretroviral therapy (HAART) improves cognition and prolongs life.
- Psychostimulants target fatigue and psychomotor retardation.

Huntington Disease (HD)

Huntington disease is an autosomal-dominant genetic disorder that results in progressively disabling cognitive, physical, and psychological functioning, ultimately resulting in death.

CLINICAL MANIFESTATIONS

- Onset: 35–50 years of age.
- Progressive dementia:
  - Dementia typically begins 1 year before or 1 year after the chorea.
  - Patients are often aware of deteriorating mentation.
- Choreiform (dancelike) movements.
- Muscular hypertonicity.
- Psychiatric manifestations include depression, psychosis, and alcoholism.
- ↑ rate of suicide.

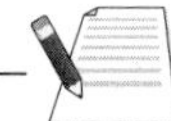

HD is caused by expanded trinucleotide (CAG) repeats. The longer the CAG repeat, the earlier the age of onset.

DIAGNOSIS

- MRI shows caudate atrophy (and sometimes cortical atrophy).
- Genetic testing.

PATHOLOGY

Trinucleotide repeat on short arm of chromosome 4.

TREATMENT

There is no effective treatment available (supportive only).

Parkinson Disease (PD)

A 46-year-old man presents with recurrent attacks of smelling strange smells and a sensation that objects appear very small (lilliputian hallucinations), followed by a temporary loss of consciousness. His wife says that he tends to smack his lips during these episodes. What is the likely diagnosis? Temporal lobe epilepsy.

- Parkinson disease is a progressive disease with prominent neuronal loss in substantia nigra, which provides dopamine to the basal ganglia, causing physical and cognitive impairment.
- Approximately 30–40% of patients with Parkinson disease develop dementia.
- Fifty percent of patients will suffer from depression.
- Occurs slightly more in men than in women.

Etiology

- Idiopathic (most common)
- Traumatic (eg, Muhammad Ali)
- Drug- or toxin-induced
- Encephalitic (as in the book/movie *Awakenings*)
- Familial (rare)

Clinical Manifestations

- Dementia symptoms resemble Alzheimer's type: Dementia rarely occurs as an initial symptom.
- Parkinsonism (bradykinesia, cogwheel rigidity, resting tremor, masklike facial expression, shuffling gait, dysarthria).

Pathology

- Loss of cells in the substantia nigra of the basal ganglia, → a ↓ in dopamine and loss of the dopaminergic tracts.
- Similar to Alzheimer disease: Senile plaques and neurofibrillary tangles, loss of neurons, and ↓ choline acetyltransferase.

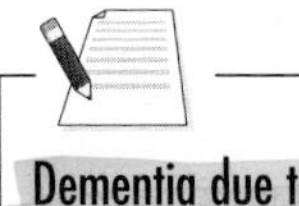

Dementia due to Parkinson disease is exacerbated by antipsychotic medications.

Creutzfeldt-Jakob Disease (CJD)

- CJD is a rapidly progressive, degenerative disease of the central nervous system (CNS) caused by accumulation of abnormal forms of prions (proteinaceous infectious particles that are normally expressed by healthy neurons of the brain).
- Affects older patients, and may be inherited, sporadic, or acquired.
- A small percentage of patients have become infected through corneal transplants.

Clinical Manifestations

- Rapidly progressive dementia 6–12 months after onset of symptoms.
- More than 90% of patients have myoclonus (sudden spasms of muscles).
- Bansal ganglia and cerebellar dysfunction is common.
- Personality changes, immature behavior, and paranoia are early signs.
- Rapid progression to stupor, coma, death in a matter of months to a few years.

Diagnosis

- Definitive: Pathological demonstration of spongiform changes of brain tissue
- Probable: The presence of both rapidly progressive dementia and periodic generalized sharp waves on electroencephalogram (EEG) plus at least two of the following clinical features:
  - Myoclonus
  - Cortical blindness
  - Ataxia, pyramidal signs, or extrapyramidal signs
  - Muscle atrophy
  - Mutism

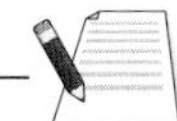

Other prion diseases include kuru, Gerstmann-Straussler syndrome, fatal familial insomnia, and bovine spongiform encephalopathy ("mad cow disease").

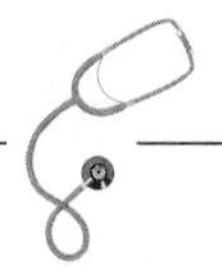

The 3 W's of NPH
Wobbly = Gait disturbance
Wet = Urinary incontinence
Wacky = Dementia

Normal Pressure Hydrocephalus (NPH)

- NPH is a potentially reversible cause of dementia.
- These patients have enlarged ventricles with ↑ cerebrospinal fluid (CSF) pressure.
- The etiology is either idiopathic or secondary to obstruction of CSF reabsorption sites due to trauma, infection, or hemorrhage.

Clinical Manifestations

Clinical triad:

- Gait disturbance: Apraxia (often appears first)
- Urinary incontinence
- Dementia (mild, insidious onset)

Treatment

- Relieve ↑ pressure with shunt.
- Of the clinical triad, dementia is least likely to improve.

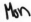

HIGH-YIELD FACTS IN

Geriatric Psychiatry

The geriatric population of the United States is projected to more than double by the year 2050, boosted in a large part by the aging Baby Boomer generation. Nearly 20% of people over the age of 55 have mental disorders outside deficits of normal aging. The suicide rate of elderly, aged 85 and older, is twice the national average.

Common diagnoses in elderly patients include mood disorders, anxiety disorders, and cognitive impairments, though many mental disorders in this population remain underreported.

NORMAL AGING

Factors associated with normal aging include:

- ↓ brain weight/enlarged ventricles and sulci
- ↓ muscle mass/↑ fat
- Impaired vision and hearing
- Minor forgetfulness (called benign senescent forgetfulness)

MAJOR DEPRESSION

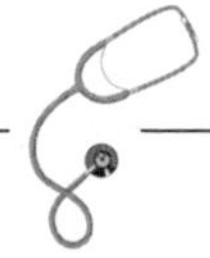

Work up an elderly patient for major depression when he or she presents with memory loss or nonspecific physical complaints.

Major depression is a common mental disorder in the geriatric population, with depressive symptoms present in 8–20% of the elderly. Depression can be associated with physical health:

- Post–myocardial infarction (MI) patients who develop depression have an ↑ rate of death.
- Stroke patients who develop depression have an ↑ rate of death during the 10 years following their stroke.
- New admits to nursing homes suffering from depression have an ↑ 1-year mortality rate.

PSEUDODEMENTIA

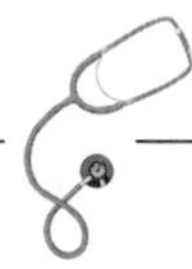

Patients with dementia are more likely to confabulate when they do not know an answer, whereas depressed patients may just say they don't know. When pressed for an answer, depressed patients will often show the capacity to answer correctly.

Symptoms of major depression in the elderly often include problems with memory and cognitive functioning. Because this clinical picture may be mistaken for dementia, it is termed *pseudodementia*.

Pseudodementia is the presence of apparent cognitive deficits in patients with major depression. Patients may appear demented. However, their symptoms are only secondary to their underlying depression, and it can be difficult to differentiate the two (see Table 8-1).

TREATMENT

- Supportive psychotherapy.
- Community resources: Senior centers, senior services, support groups, etc.
- Low-dose antidepressant medication (selective serotonin reuptake inhibitors [SSRIs] have the fewest side effects and are generally preferable to tricyclic antidepressants [TCAs] or monoamine oxidase [MAO] inhibitors).
- If using TCAs in elderly patients, nortriptyline is favored because it has the fewest anticholinergic side effects.

TABLE 8-1. Dementia Versus Pseudodementia (Depression)

DEMENTIA	PSEUDODEMENTIA (DEPRESSION)
Onset is insidious.	Onset is more acute.
Sundowning is common (↑ confusion at night).	Sundowning is uncommon.
Will guess at answers (confabulate).	Often answers "I don't know."
Patient is unaware of problems.	Patient is aware of problems.
Cognitive deficits do not improve with antidepressant treatment.	Cognitive deficits improve with antidepressants.

- Mirtazapine can ↑ appetite and is also sedating; it is often dosed at bedtime for depressed patients who also suffer from ↓ appetite and sleep disturbances.
- Methylphenidate can be used at low doses as an adjunct to antidepressants for patients with psychomotor retardation; however, it may cause insomnia if given in the afternoon or evening. Also be aware of arrhythmia risks in cardiac patients.
- Electroconvulsive therapy (ECT) may be used in place of antidepressants (safe and effective in the elderly).

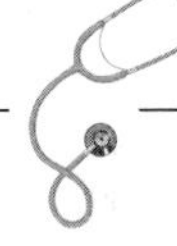

The elderly are very sensitive to side effects of antidepressant medications, particularly anticholinergics.

Mrs. Brennan is a 72-year-old Caucasian woman who considers herself to be in good health. She goes out to lunch with friends three times a week and looks forward to her Saturday bridge games at the local senior center. Unfortunately, her husband has suffered from years of ill health, including five myocardial infarctions and a serious stroke last year that left him barely able to walk. You are a geriatric psychiatrist who has been treating Mrs. Brennan's husband for depression that began after his last stroke. Mrs. Brennan always comes along to appointments so that she can stay informed about her husband's medical care.

You become concerned when your patient uncharacteristically misses an appointment and does not return your phone message. Finally, a month later, you are surprised to see Mrs. Brennan walk into your office alone. She enters the room slowly, and you notice that she has lost some weight since you last saw her.

She sits down but does not make eye contact. Finally, she begins to talk in a soft, monotone voice, explaining that her husband had another bad stroke last month and was moved to a hospice facility, where he passed away 2 weeks ago. She begins to cry, and you hand her some tissues. The two of you talk some more about her husband's death and how she is coping with it. She reports that her daughter visits her frequently and has invited her to spend the weekends with her.

Although Mrs. Brennan reports that she feels "down," she reports that she is making an effort to go on with her life because that is what her husband would

(continued)

have wanted. She says that she went out to lunch with her friends this week and adds that they are very supportive. Mrs. Brennan also reports that it is difficult for her to realize that her husband is no longer there and says that she has heard his voice calling her a couple of times this week. As she leaves your office, you tell her she is welcome to come back whenever she wants.

Is Mrs. Brennan having a normal grief reaction?

Yes, Mrs. Brennan is going through a normal grieving process, also known as bereavement. Although she displays some symptoms suggestive of depression (psychomotor retardation, depressed mood), and reports the presence of auditory hallucinations (her husband's voice), these symptoms are commonly encountered in bereavement and are considered a normal reaction to her sudden loss.

Three months later, you receive a phone call from Mrs. Brennan's daughter, who expresses concern about her mother. She tells you that her mother has to be urged to shower, wear clean clothes, and eat regularly. Mrs. Brennan has stopped participating in her bridge group and has not been out with her friends in many weeks. The daughter also worries about Mrs. Brennan's increasing forgetfulness and memory problems. She asks if she can bring her in for an appointment with you. You agree immediately and schedule Mrs. Brennan the next day.

Mrs. Brennan enters your office with her daughter by her side. She is dressed in a wrinkled pantsuit and is wearing scuffed shoes. Her hair is clean but lies limply against her head. She appears much thinner than the last time you saw her. Her eyes are downcast, and she appears sad. You try to engage her in conversation, but her answers to your questions are soft and short. When you do an assessment of her memory, you note that she answers basic questions with "I don't know" and scores poorly on mini-mental questions.

What is Mrs. Brennan's most likely diagnosis now?

Mrs. Brennan is most likely suffering from depression. Her symptoms now fulfill criteria for major depressive disorder and have been present for over 2 months. Since her memory problems began after she began experiencing depressive symptoms, these are most likely secondary to depression. When this occurs, it is referred to as pseudodementia. If this is the case, as her depression is treated, her memory deficits will improve.

What are possible treatment options for Mrs. Brennan?

Supportive psychotherapy and a medication trial of a low-dose SSRI would be excellent first-line treatments. In addition, you suggest to Mrs. Brennan and her daughter to consider visiting her local senior center to learn what kinds of services she might benefit from.

BEREAVEMENT

In 1969, Elisabeth Kübler-Ross, MD, published a seminal book in the field of palliative care, called *On Death and Dying*. In it, she proposed a model of bereavement, the Five Stages of Grief.

- **Denial:** *"This isn't happening to me. I don't feel sick."*
- **Anger:** *"It's my ex-husband's fault for smoking around me all those years!"*
- **Bargaining:** *"Maybe if I exercise and improve my diet, I'll get better."*
- **Depression:** *"There's no hope for a cure. I will die of this cancer."*
- **Acceptance:** *"I may have cancer, but I've always been a fighter—why stop now?"*

People may not experience all of the stages, or they may go through them in a different order. Grief is often a very individualized experience, and there is no "correct" way to mourn a loss. However, it is important to be able to distinguish normal grief reactions from unhealthy, pathological ones.

- **Normal grief** may involve many intense feelings, including guilt and sadness, sleep disturbances, appetite changes, and illusions (not always pathological in some cultures). These feelings generally abate within 6 months of the loss, and the patient's ability to function appropriately in their life is preserved.
- **Complicated/prolonged grief** persists for at least 6 months and includes at least four of these eight symptoms:
  1. Difficulty moving on with life
  2. Numbness/detachment
  3. Bitterness
  4. Feeling that life is empty without the deceased
  5. Trouble accepting the loss
  6. Feeling that the future holds no meaning without the deceased
  7. Agitation
  8. Difficulty trusting others since the loss
- **Bereavement-associated depression** is essentially major depression that began with a concrete death or loss in the patient's life. It is quite difficult to distinguish between depression and complicated grief, since many symptoms are similar.
  - Look for generalized feelings of hopelessness, helplessness, severe guilt and worthlessness, and suicidal ideation, in addition to complicated grief symptoms.
  - Treatment for depression is recommended in patients who have 2 straight weeks of depressive symptoms 6–8 weeks after the precipitating loss.

SUBSTANCE ABUSE

- Nearly half of the 65+-year-old population drinks alcohol, and up to 15% of those people may experience adverse health events from the amount of alcohol they use or from its interaction with medications and impact on chronic disease processes.
- Age-related effects of alcohol:
  - ↓ alcohol dehydrogenase can → higher blood alcohol levels (BALs) with fewer drinks as compared to younger adults
  - ↑ central nervous system sensitivity to alcohol

TABLE 8-2. **Alcohol and Medication Interactions**

Medication	Result of Concurrent Alcohol Use
H_2 blockers	Higher BALs
Benzodiazepines, tricyclics, narcotics, barbiturates, antihistamines	↑ sedation
Aspirin, NSAIDs	Prolonged bleeding time Irritation of gastric lining
Metronidazole, sulfonamides, long-acting hypoglycemics	Nausea and vomiting
Reserpine, nitroglycerin, hydralazine	↑ risk of hypotension
Acetaminophen, isoniazid, phenylbutazone	↑ hepatotoxicity
Antihypertensives, antidiabetics, ulcer drugs, gout medications	Worsen underlying disease

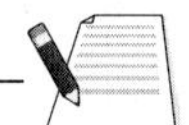

The most common psychiatric disorder in the elderly is major depressive disorder.

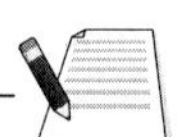

White elderly males have the highest rate of **successful** suicides.

- Chronic medical conditions worsened by alcohol:
  - Liver diseases (cirrhosis, hepatitis)
  - Gastrointestinal (GI) diseases (GI bleeding, gastric reflux, ulcer)
  - Cardiovascular diseases (hypertension, heart failure)
  - Metabolic/endocrine diseases (gout, diabetes)
  - Mental disorders (depression, anxiety)
- Alcohol and medication interactions: See Table 8-2.

PSYCHIATRIC MANIFESTATIONS OF DEMENTIA

Behavioral symptoms are quite common in patients with dementia, and often the source of many psychosocial problems surrounding the care of dementia patients. Agitation and aggression can be distressing and dangerous for caregivers, as well as unsafe for patients. Behavioral disinhibition is fairly common in dementias and causes patients to act in ways that are quite unlike their typical behaviors (stripping off clothes in public, sexualized behavior, cursing).

- Mood disorders:
  - Difficult to diagnose in a patient with confirmed dementia.
  - Dementia patients may display many symptoms of depression that are merely natural manifestations of their disease.
  - Mood and affect are often poor diagnostic indicators in patients with moderate to severe cognitive impairment.
- Aggression:
  - May be provoked by the patient's confusion in the setting of cognitive, memory, and language deficits
  - May be provoked by hallucinations or delusions
- Psychosis:
  - Delusions are reported in up to 70% of Alzheimer patients.
  - Hallucinations can be seen in up to 33% of dementia patients.

- In the setting of a dementia, most hallucinations are visual.
- If hallucinations do not bother the patient or interfere with caring for the patient, pharmacotherapy is unnecessary.

> Visual hallucinations early in dementia suggest a diagnosis of dementia with Lewy bodies. Do not give these patients antipsychotics.

TREATMENT

Behavioral and environmental treatments for behavioral symptoms are much preferred in the elderly. Pharmacological methods are appropriate in the setting of potentially harmful behaviors, but care must be taken in dosing, duration of treatment, and interactions with other medications.

- Nonpharmacological treatments:
  - Music, art, exercise, and pet therapy.
  - Strict daily schedules to minimize changes in routine.
  - Continual reorientation of patient.
  - Reduce stimuli (quiet living environments).
  - Surround patient with familiar objects (family photos, a favorite quilt, etc).
- Pharmacological treatments:
  - Antipsychotics:
    - Limited efficacy and ↑ mortality.
    - Try olanzapine (Zyprexa) or quetiapine (Seroquel) in patients with severe symptoms.
    - Can also use short-term haloperidol (Haldol) or risperidone (Risperdal).
  - Anxiolytics:
    - Anxiety symptoms may be due to unrecognized depression and respond well to an SSRI.
    - Reserve benzodiazepines for very short-term, acute episodes and remember to watch for paradoxical agitation.
  - Mood stabilizers: Most commonly used are valproic acid, carbamazepine, and lamotrigine; however, there are few studies on their effectiveness in the elderly.

SLEEP DISTURBANCES

The incidence of sleep disorders ↑ with aging. Elderly people often report difficulty sleeping, daytime drowsiness, and daytime napping.

- Outside of normal changes associated with aging (see Table 8-3), causes of sleep disturbances may include general medical conditions, drug/alcohol use, social stressors, and medications.
- Patients with movement disorders (Parkinson disease, progressive supranuclear palsy) have shallow sleep and may be more restless at night because of trouble turning in bed.
- Restless leg movements during sleep, often due to a dopamine imbalance, are called periodic leg movements (PLMs).
- Nonpharmacological treatment approaches should be tried first (alcohol cessation, ↑ daily structure, elimination of daytime naps, treatment of underlying medical conditions that may be exacerbating sleep problems).
- Sedative-hypnotic drugs are more likely to cause side effects when used by the elderly (memory impairment, ataxia, paradoxical excitement, and rebound insomnia).

TABLE 8-3. Normal Sleep Changes in Geriatric Patients

Rapid eye movement (REM) sleep	↓ REM latency and ↓ total REM
Non-REM sleep	↑ amounts of stage 1 and 2 sleep, ↓ amounts of stage 3 and 4 sleep (deep sleep)
Sleep efficiency	↓ (frequent nocturnal awakenings)
Amount of total sleep	↓
Sleep cycle	Sleep cycle advances (earlier to bed, earlier to rise)

- If sedative-hypnotics must be prescribed, medications such as hydroxyzine (Vistaril) or trazodone are safer than the more sedating benzodiazepines.

OTHER ISSUES

Restraints

- In nonemergency situations, restraints should be used as a last resort and the patient should be reassessed at regular intervals.
- Patient safety, health, and well-being should be the most important concern in the matter of restraint use.

Medications

- Many older people are on multiple medications.
- They suffer from more side effects because of ↓ lean body mass and impaired liver and kidney function.
- When confronted with a new symptom in an elderly patient on multiple medications, always try to remove a medication before adding one.

Elder Abuse

- Types: Physical abuse, psychological abuse (threats, insults, etc), neglect (withholding of care), exploitation (misuse of finances), and rarely sexual abuse.
- Ten percent of all people > 65 years old; underreported by victims.
- Perpetrator is usually a caregiver who lives with the victim.

Nursing Homes

- Provide care and rehabilitation for chronically ill and impaired patients as well as for patients who are in need of short-term care before returning to their prior living arrangements.
- Approximately half the patients stay on permanently, and half are discharged after only a few months.

HIGH-YIELD FACTS IN

Psychiatric Disorders in Children

PSYCHIATRIC EXAMINATION OF A CHILD

Sources of Information

In child psychiatry, it is important to consult multiple sources when gathering information:

- Child
- Parent/caregiver
- Teachers and coaches
- Pediatrician
- Child welfare/juvenile justice system (if relevant)

Methods of Gathering Information

- **Diagnostic play sessions:** Involve having the child reveal their internal states and experiences through the use of *play*, *storytelling*, or *drawing*.
- **Classroom observation:** Can help provide greater insight into child's functioning in school.
- **Formal neuropsychological testing:** Can help clarify diagnoses by quantitatively assessing a child's strengths and weaknesses by examination of intelligence quotient (IQ); language and visual-motor skills; and memory, attention, and organizational abilities.
- **Kaufman Assessment Battery for Children (K-ABC):** Intelligence test for ages 2–12.
- **Wechsler Intelligence Scale for Children–Revised (WISC-R):** Determines IQ for ages 6–16.

MENTAL RETARDATION (MR)

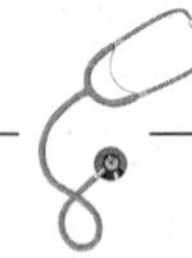

A diagnosis of MR cannot be made with just a low IQ. Deficits in adaptive skills must also be present.

Intellectual disability is currently the preferred term for the disability historically referred to as mental retardation, but mental retardation is still defined by the *Diagnostic and Statistical Manual of Mental Disorders*, 4th ed., Text Revision (DSM-IV-TR) as:

- Significantly subaverage intellectual functioning with an IQ of ≤ 70.
- Deficits in adaptive skills appropriate for the age group.
- Onset must be before the age of 18.

Epidemiology

- Affects 1–3% of the population.
- Approximately 85% of mentally retarded are *mild* cases.
- Males are affected 1.5 times as often as females.

Subclassifications

Type of MR	Definition	Approx % of MR
Profound	IQ < 25	1–2%
Severe	IQ 25–40	3–4%
Moderate	IQ 40–55	10%
Mild	IQ 55–70	85%

TABLE 9-1. Causes of Mental Retardation

CAUSE	EXAMPLES
Genetic	**Down syndrome:** Trisomy 21 (1/700 live births) **Fragile X syndrome:** Involves mutation of X chromosome, second most common cause of retardation, M > F Others: Phenylketonuria, familial mental retardation, Prader-Willi syndrome, Williams syndrome, Angelman syndrome, tuberous sclerosis
Prenatal	Infection and toxins **(TORCH):** ▪ **T**oxoplasmosis ▪ **O**ther (syphilis, AIDS, alcohol/illicit drugs) ▪ **R**ubella (German measles) ▪ **C**ytomegalovirus (CMV) ▪ **H**erpes simplex
Perinatal	Anoxia, prematurity, birth trauma, meningitis, hyperbilirubinemia
Postnatal	Hypothyroidism, malnutrition, toxin exposure, trauma, psychosocial causes

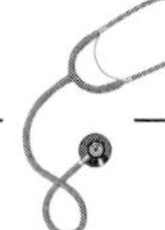

Prader-Willi syndrome patients typically have mental retardation, obesity, hypogonadism, and almond-shaped eyes.

CAUSES

As much as 50% of MR has no identifiable cause, and other causes include genetic, prenatal, perinatal, and postnatal conditions (see Table 9-1).

LEARNING DISORDERS

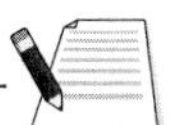

The most common inherited form of mental retardation is fragile X syndrome, resulting from an *FMR-1* gene defect. Patients with fragile X syndrome usually exhibit autistic characteristics, delayed speech, motor delay, and sensory deficits. Males have large testicles.

Learning disorders are defined by the DSM-IV as achievement in reading, mathematics, or written expression that is significantly lower than expected for chronological age, level of education, and level of intelligence.

- Learning disorders affect academic achievement or daily activities.
- Cannot be explained by sensory deficits, poor teaching, or cultural factors.
- Are often due to deficits in cognitive processing (abnormal attention, memory, visual perception, etc).

EPIDEMIOLOGY

- **Reading disorder:**
  - Most common of learning disorders.
  - Affects 4–10% of school-age children.
  - Boys may be affected more than girls.
- **Mathematics disorder:**
  - Affects 1% of school-age children.
  - Male-to-female ratio may be more equal.
- **Disorder of written expression:**
  - Affects 6% of school-age children.
  - Male-to-female ratio unknown.

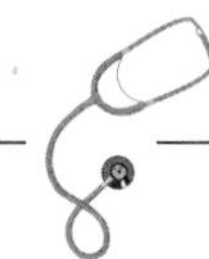

Always rule out sensory deficits before diagnosing learning disorders.

Etiology

Learning disorders may be caused by genetic factors, abnormal development, perinatal injury, and neurological or medical conditions.

Treatment

Remedial education tailored to the child's specific needs.

DISRUPTIVE BEHAVIOR DISORDERS

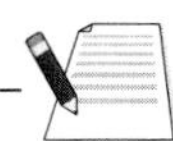

Unlike conduct disorder, ODD does not involve physical aggression or violation of the basic rights of others.

Some defiance is developmentally appropriate for children. Disruptive behavior disorders include symptoms that result in impairment in social and/or academic function and include oppositional defiant disorder and conduct disorder.

Oppositional Defiant Disorder (ODD)

Diagnosis and DSM-IV Criteria

At least 6 months of negativistic, hostile, and defiant behavior during which at least four of the following have been present:

1. Frequent loss of temper
2. Arguments with adults
3. Defying adults' rules
4. Deliberately annoying people
5. Easily annoyed
6. Anger and resentment
7. Spitefulness
8. Blaming others for mistakes or misbehaviors

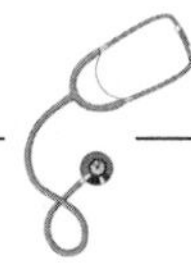

In cases of kids who have no difficulties getting along with their peers but will not comply with expectations from parents or teachers, *think: oppositional defiant disorder (ODD).*

Epidemiology

- Prevalence: Reports range from 2% to 16%.
- Can begin as early as age 3, usually observed by age 8.
- Onset before puberty is more common in boys; onset after puberty equal in boys and girls.
- ↑ incidence of comorbid substance abuse, mood disorders, and attention deficit/hyperactivity disorder (ADHD).
- Twenty-five percent of cases will no longer meet criteria in later years; in persistent cases, may progress to conduct disorder.

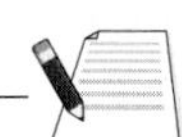

Cruelty to animals may be a hint at **conduct disorder.**

Treatment

Treatment should involve individual psychotherapy that focuses on behavior modification and problem-solving skills as well as include family involvement with a focus on parent management skills training.

Conduct Disorder

Conduct disorder is the most serious disruptive behavior disorder, and it is the clinical term that captures very "bad boys" and "bad girls."

Diagnosis and DSM-IV Criteria

A persistent pattern of behavior in which the basic rights of others or social norms are violated, as evidenced by the presence of at least 3 out of 15 described behaviors during the past year. The behaviors are grouped within the following categories:

1. Aggression toward people and animals
2. Destruction of property
3. Deceitfulness or theft
4. Serious violations of rules

Children with conduct disorder have a higher risk of substance abuse and making suicidal gestures and attempts.

> **Differences between boys and girls with conduct disorder:**
> **Boys: Higher risk of fighting, stealing, fire-setting, vandalism**
> **Girls: Higher risk of lying, running away, sexually acting out**

Epidemiology

- Prevalence: 1–10%.
- Four to 12 times more common in boys.
- Risk factors: Punitive parenting, psychosocial adversity, history of being abused, biological predisposition.
- High incidence of comorbid ADHD (up to 70%) and learning disorders.
- ↑ risk for mood disorders, substance abuse, and criminal behavior in adulthood.
- Up to 40% will go on to develop antisocial personality disorder in adulthood.

Treatment

- A multimodal treatment approach with family and community involvement is most effective.
- Consistent rules and consequences are important in reducing problematic behaviors.
- Medications can be a useful adjunct if aggression is present (antipsychotics, mood stabilizers, and selective serotonin reuptake inhibitors [SSRIs]).

An 8-year-old girl is referred for evaluation because of academic and behavior problems at school and at home that have been going on for about a year. The girl's mother reports that when she is at home, she appears to be "driven by a motor." She is also often forgetful and loses things regularly.

Her teacher was interviewed and reported that the girl has been making a lot of careless mistakes in her assignments and constantly fidgets in her seat, sometimes appearing restless during tests. She also has trouble waiting her turn and refraining from blurting out answers and interrupting the class. The teacher is especially concerned about these behaviors because she believes the girl is generally intelligent and a "good girl."

The girl's soccer coach reported that the child doesn't always listen to directions during practice and has problems paying attention during games.

(continued)

Autistic Disorder

DSM-IV-TR Diagnosis

At least six symptoms must be present by age 3, with at least two from (1) and least one from (2) and (3):

1. **Problems with social interaction:** Impairment in nonverbal behaviors, lack of peer relationships, lack of interest in sharing enjoyment with others, lack of social/emotional reciprocity
2. **Impairments in communication:** Delayed speech, inability to hold conversations, repetitive or stereotyped use of language, lack of make-believe and imitative play
3. **Repetitive and stereotyped patterns of behavior and activities:** Narrowed interests, inflexible adherence to rituals, repetitive motor mannerisms (hand flapping), preoccupation with parts of objects

Abnormalities in functioning must be present by age 3. The condition cannot be better accounted for by Rett disorder or childhood disintegrative disorder.

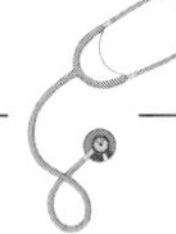

In evaluating a toddler who shows no interest or does not speak unless spoken to directly, it is important to order a hearing test before making a diagnosis of autism.

Epidemiology

- There has been a recent ↑ in reported prevalence, but this could be related to changes in definition, as well as ↑ awareness and recognition of the condition.
- Estimates of incidence range from 1 in 1000 children to 1 in 100.
- Boys are affected three to four times more than girls.
- Seventy percent of individuals with autism meet criteria for mental retardation (IQ < 70).
- Association with fragile X syndrome, tuberous sclerosis, and seizures.

Etiology

The etiology of autism is multifactorial, including:

- Prenatal neurological insults (from infections, drugs, etc).
- Genetic factors (siblings of affected persons are at a greater than 22-fold risk of autism than the general population).
- Immunological and biochemical factors (individuals with autism may have higher peripheral serotonin levels), ↑ head size, persistent primitive reflexes, and abnormalities on electrocardiographic (EEG) testing.

Prognosis and Treatment

Prognosis is variable, but the two most important predictors of adult outcome are level of intellectual functioning and communicative competence. There is no cure for autism, but various treatments are used to help manage symptoms and improve basic social, communicative, and cognitive skills:

- Remedial education (ideally on an intensive and continuous basis).
- Behavioral therapy.
- Antipsychotic medications (to help control aggression, hyperactivity, and mood lability).
- Consider antidepressants or stimulants if other symptoms warrant them.

Asperger Disorder

Diagnosis and DSM-IV Criteria

This condition is characterized by the same impairments seen in autism involving social interaction and restricted or stereotyped interests and behaviors, but it differs from autism in that there is no clinically significant delay in spoken or receptive language, cognitive development, self-help skills, or curiosity about the environment.

> **Unlike autistic disorder, children with Asperger disorder have normal language acquisition and cognitive development.**

Epidemiology

- Incidence is unknown.
- More common in boys than in girls.
- Social interaction is often characterized by a "professorial" or "pedantic" style.
- Social difficulties often → chronic frustration and ↑ risk for depression in adolescence.

Etiology

Unknown etiology but may involve genetic, infectious, or perinatal factors as in autism.

Treatment

- Supportive treatment as used with autism.
- Preservation of verbal abilities will allow for more benefit from social skills training and behavioral modification techniques.

Rett Disorder

- Rett disorder is characterized by normal physical and psychomotor development during the first 5 months after birth, followed by a decreasing rate of head growth and loss of previously learned purposeful hand skills between ages 5 and 30 months.
- These children will then develop stereotyped hand movements (hand wringing, hand washing), impaired language and psychomotor retardation, and problems with gait or trunk movements.

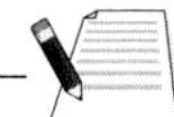

> **In Rett disorder, cognitive development never progresses beyond that of the first year of life.**

Features

- Onset between age 5 and 48 months.
- Seen in girls predominantly; boys have variable phenotype, and it is most likely lethal in utero for males.
- Rare, between 1 in 15,000 and 1 in 22,000 females.
- Genetic testing is available.
- EEG is frequently abnormal, and seizures are common.
- Associated with *MECP2* gene mutation on X chromosome.
- Patients may become nonambulatory due to motor problems and scoliosis.
- ↑ risk of sudden death.
- **Treatment:** Supportive.

Childhood Disintegrative Disorder

In this disorder, there is normal development in the first 2 years of life, including communication, social relationships, play, and adaptive behavior, but there is loss of previously acquired skills before age 10 years in at least two of these areas: language, social skills or adaptive behavior, bowel or bladder control, play, motor skills; and in at least two of these areas: impaired social interaction, impaired communication, restricted, repetitive, stereotyped behaviors, and interests.

Features

- Onset after age 2 years, usually between ages 3 and 4 years, must be before 10 years.
- Four to eight times higher incidence in boys than girls.
- Rare, maybe 1 in 100,000 children.
- Etiology is unknown.
- High rates of EEG abnormality and seizure disorder.
- Has been associated with various general medical conditions (eg, Landau-Kleffner syndrome, neurolipidoses, mitochondrial deficits, metachromatic leukodystrophy, CNS infection, etc).
- **Treatment:** Supportive, with a focus on helping child relearn basic skills.

In contrast to Rett disorder, head growth does not slow, and the unusual hand movements are not present in childhood disintegrative disorder.

TOURETTE DISORDER

Tics are sudden, repetitive, nonrhythmic, stereotyped involuntary movements or vocalizations. Tourette disorder is the most severe tic disorder and is characterized by multiple daily motor and one or more vocal tics with onset before age 18 years. Vocal tics may first appear many years after the motor tics. The most common **motor tics** involve the face and head, such as blinking of the eyes. Examples of **vocal tics** include:

- *Coprolalia*—repetitive speaking of obscene words (uncommon in children)
- *Echolalia*—exact repetition of words

Diagnosis and DSM-IV Criteria

- Multiple motor and one or more vocal tics (both must be present at some time during illness, but not necessarily concurrently) that are not attributable to CNS disease (ie, Huntington disease or postviral encephalopathies).
- Onset prior to age 18 years.
- Tics occur many times a day, almost every day for > 1 year (no tic-free period > 3 months).
- Change in anatomic location and character of tics over time.
- Both motor and vocal tics must be present to diagnose Tourette disorder.

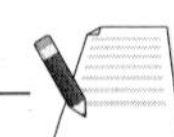

Tic disorders are one of the few psychiatric disorders in which a diagnosis can be given without symptoms causing significant distress.

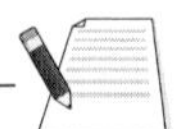

Psychopharmacology is treatment of choice for Tourette disorder.

Epidemiology

- Transient tic behaviors: common in children, occurs in 4–24% of school-age children.
- Tourette disorder: Estimates are between 5 and 300 per 10,000.
- Boys > girls.

- Waxing/waning course, tic episodes occur in bouts, which also tend to cluster.
- Symptoms peak in severity between ages 8 and 12 years, decreasing with puberty.
- One-half to two-thirds experience marked reduction of symptoms by their late teens, with one-third to one-half becoming virtually asymptomatic in adulthood.
- High comorbidity with obsessive-compulsive disorder (40%) and ADHD (50%).

Etiology

- Genetic factors: 50% concordance rate in monozygotic versus 10% in dizygotic twins.
- Perinatal factors: Potential risk factors include severity of maternal life stress during pregnancy, severe nausea and/or vomiting during first trimester, prematurity, or low birth weight.
- Neurochemical factors: Impaired regulation of **dopamine** in the caudate nucleus (and possibly impaired regulation of endogenous opiates and the noradrenergic system).
- Postinfectious autoimmune factors: Circumstantial evidence linking group A beta-hemolytic streptococcal infection to development of some tic and obsessive-compulsive disorders (OCDs).
- Psychological factors: Symptom exacerbations follow stressful life events, fatigue, extremes of temperature, and external stimuli.

Treatment

- Educational and supportive interventions: Create realistic expectations, supportive classroom environments.
- Psychological: Supportive therapy, behavioral therapy.
- Pharmacological:
  - Utilized when tics become a source of impairment.
  - Atypical neuroleptics (risperidone), alpha-2 agonists (clonidine, guanfacine).
  - Typical neuroleptics (haloperidol, pimozide) for severe cases.
  - Use of stimulants is controversial in ADHD associated with tic disorder, due to concern for exacerbation of tics.
  - OCD patients with comorbid tics have good response to SSRI augmentation of antipsychotics.

ELIMINATION DISORDERS

Urinary continence is normally established before age 4. Bowel control is normally achieved by the age of 4. Incontinence can result in rejection by peers and impairment of social development.

Diagnosis

- **Enuresis:** Involuntary voiding of urine (bed-wetting) after age 5 (at least twice a week for at least 3 consecutive months or with marked impairment). Rule out infections, diabetes, seizures.
- **Encopresis:** Involuntary or intentional passage of feces in inappropriate places by age 4 (at least once a month for at least 3 months). Rule out

metabolic abnormalities (hypothyroidism), lower gastrointestinal problems (anal fissure, inflammatory bowel disease), and dietary factors.

- Distinguish between primary (never established continence) versus secondary (continence achieved for a period and then lost).

EPIDEMIOLOGY

- Enuresis: 5% of 5-year-old children.
- Encopresis: 1% of 5-year-old children.
- Boys > girls.
- Prevalence ↓ with age.
- May be associated with other psychiatric conditions, such as conduct disorder.

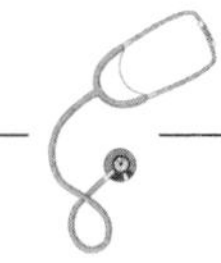

The great majority of cases of enuresis spontaneously remit by age 7.

ETIOLOGY

- Genetic predisposition
- Psychosocial stressors (especially with secondary incontinence)
- Eneuresis: Small bladder or low nocturnal levels of antidiuretic hormone
- Encopresis: Lack of sphincter control, constipation with overflow incontinence (responsible for 75% of cases)

TREATMENT

- Take into account the high spontaneous remission rates.
- Psychoeducation, psychotherapy, family therapy, and behavioral therapy.
- Enuresis: Behavior modification (ie, bell and pad method—buzzer that wakes child up when sensor detects wetness), antidiuretics (DDAVP), or tricyclic antidepressants (such as imipramine).
- Encopresis: Initial bowel catharsis followed by stool softeners (if etiology is constipation).

OTHER CHILDHOOD DISORDERS

Selective Mutism

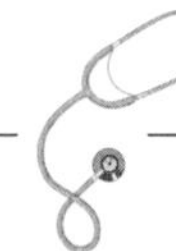

Separation anxiety is often age appropriate from 7 months to 6 years of age so is usually not diagnosed until after age 6 years.

Selective mutism is a rare condition that occurs more commonly in girls than in boys, characterized by refusal to speak in certain situations (such as in school) for at least 1 month, despite the ability to comprehend and use language.

- Onset is usually around age 2–5, although it is often not noticed until time of entry into school.
- Treatment includes psychotherapy, behavior therapy, and management of anxiety.

Stranger anxiety, the distress that children experience when with unfamiliar faces, usually peaks around 8–12 months of age.

Separation Anxiety Disorder

Separation anxiety disorder involves excessive fear for ≥ 4 weeks of leaving one's parents or other major attachment figures.

- Children with this disorder may refuse (or complain of physical symptoms to avoid) going to school or sleeping alone, and they may report physical symptoms.

- When forced to separate, they become extremely distressed and may worry excessively about losing their parents forever.
- Separation anxiety disorder affects up to 4% of school-age children, occurs equally in boys and girls, and may be preceded by a stressful life event.
- Parents are often afflicted with anxiety disorders and may express excessive concern about their children.
- Treatment involves family therapy, cognitive behavioral therapy, and low-dose antidepressants.

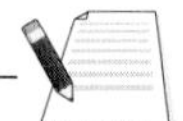

Childhood separation anxiety disorder may be a risk factor for the development of panic disorder or agoraphobia as an adolescent or adult.

Child Abuse

Child abuse includes physical abuse, emotional abuse, sexual abuse, and neglect.

- Doctors are legally required to report all cases of suspected child abuse to appropriate social service agencies.
- The majority of substantiated child abuse cases are cases of neglect.
- Adults who were abused as children have an ↑ risk of developing anxiety disorders, depressive disorders, dissociative disorders, self-destructive behaviors, substance abuse disorders, and posttraumatic stress disorder.
- They also have an ↑ risk of subsequently abusing their own children.
- Sexual abuse:
  - Fifteen to twenty-five percent of women and 5–15% of men report having been *sexually* abused as children.
  - The victim of sexual abuse is more commonly female, and the perpetrator is more commonly male and usually someone who knows the child.
  - Children are most at risk of sexual abuse between the ages of 7 and 13.
  - **Evidence of sexual abuse in a child:**
    - Sexually transmitted diseases
    - Anal or genital trauma
    - Knowledge about specific sexual acts (inappropriate for age)
    - Initiation of sexual activity with others
    - Sexual play with dolls (inappropriate for age)

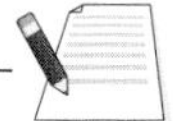

Alcohol is the most common drug of abuse by adolescents, followed by cannabis.

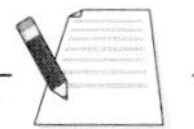

A child's parent is the most common perpetrator in substantiated child abuse cases.

NOTES

HIGH-YIELD FACTS IN

Dissociative Disorders

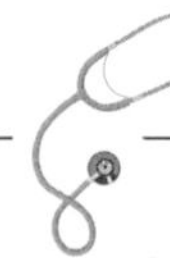

Features of dissociative disorders, such as amnesia and feelings of detachment, can come on gradually or suddenly, and they can be temporary or chronic. Dissociative responses are common in stressful and traumatic events.

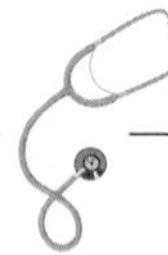

Patients with dissociative amnesia are often unable to recall common personal information but able to remember obscure details. This is opposite to the type of memory loss usually found in dementia.

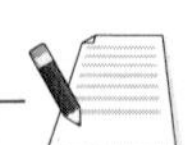

Loss of identity (such as in dissociative fugue) is not typically seen in transient global amnesia. A patient with transient global amnesia will have difficultly recalling recent events, while memory for more temporally distant events, including his or her identity, remain intact.

DEFINITION

Dissociative disorders are defined by a loss of memory (amnesia), identity, or sense of self (the normal integration of thoughts, behaviors, perceptions, feelings, and memory into a unique identity).

- Dissociative disorders have long been controversial in psychiatry.
- Dissociative disorders are often thought to be related to trauma or abuse during childhood or severe trauma as an adult.
- The neurotransmitters glutamate and norepinephrine may also be involved.
- Some argue that the more severe of these disorders are misdiagnosed personality disorders (borderline personality disorder) or are volitional.
- *Diagnostic and Statistical Manual of Mental Disorders*, 4th ed., Text Revision (DSM-IV-TR) dissociative disorders include:
  - Dissociative amnesia
  - Dissociative fugue
  - Dissociative identity disorder (previously known as multiple personality disorder)
  - Depersonalization disorder
  - Dissociative disorder not otherwise specified (NOS)

DISSOCIATIVE AMNESIA

- The diagnosis of dissociative amnesia requires that amnesia be the only dissociative symptom present.
- Patients with this disorder very often retain new memory formation and can have large periods of time that are forgotten.

Diagnosis and DSM-IV Criteria

- At least one episode of inability to recall important personal information, usually involving a traumatic or stressful event.
- The amnesia cannot be explained by ordinary forgetfulness.
- Symptoms cause significant distress or impairment in daily functioning and cannot be explained by another disorder, including traumatic brain injury, medical condition, or substance use.

Epidemiology

- Most common dissociative disorder
- More common in women than men
- More common in younger than older adults
- ↑ incidence of comorbid major depression and anxiety disorders

Course and Prognosis

Many acute cases abruptly return to normal after minutes to days. Recurrences are uncommon.

Treatment

- Most important is the establishment of the patient's safety.
- Psychotherapy is the mainstay of treatment.

- No specific psychopharmacology is approved for amnesia, but specific symptoms can be targeted, which could help alleviate barriers to treatment.
- Hypnosis or administration of sodium amobarbital or lorazepam (Ativan) during the interview have been used historically and may be useful to help some patients talk more freely.

A 22-year-old Caucasian woman is found by a couple, walking alone at night. Concerned about her wandering around in an isolated area of town, the couple stops and asks her if she needs any help. She stares at them and says that she is fine but is unable to provide her name or any contact information. She was found holding a bus ticket that suggested she had traveled from a nearby state. The couple calls an ambulance, and she is taken to a nearby emergency room where she is identified as Ms. Jane Doe.

Upon examination, Ms. Doe shows no signs of trauma. Diagnostic tests, including imaging, toxicology, and electroencephalogram, return normal. Although she is unable to provide any personal information, her purse contains a driver's license identifying her as Mary Clark, and a cell phone is found showing multiple missed calls. With the intention of communicating with close family members, you call a number identified as "mom," and you learn that her family has been worried about her whereabouts since 2 days ago, when they received a call that she had not arrived at work. Her mother reports that she had contacted the local police department to file a missing person complaint.

Ms. Clark's mother reports that her daughter has no prior psychiatric history or any medical conditions. When asked about recent stressors, she says that her daughter has been concerned about being laid off from work. Her mother reports that she will be taking the next flight available to be at her daughter's side.

What is this patient's diagnosis?

The patient's diagnosis is consistent with dissociative fugue. Ms. Clark presented with amnesia about personal identity after a sudden, unexpected travel away from home. This usually occurs after experiencing overwhelming stress or traumatic loss. Although some patients with dissociative fugue assume a new identity, most do not. It is important to consider medical conditions, such as partial complex seizures, substance use, dissociative identity disorder, depersonalization disorder, acute stress disorder, and malingering in the differential diagnosis.

What is the recommended treatment?

Most dissociative fugue episodes resolve in a few hours to a few days. However, Ms. Clark would benefit from a psychotherapeutic approach to help her cope with psychosocial stressors and to increase awareness of her reactions and feelings toward stressful situations. If the dissociative state persists, hypnosis might be effective in retrieving memories and making these available to consciousness. Although their use in dissociative fugue is controversial, an intravenous benzodiazepine, sodium amobarbital, or other short-acting sedatives might be used to elicit memories.

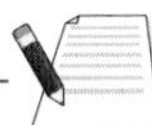

Dissociative amnesia refers to a disruption in the continuity of a person's memory. Patients with dissociative amnesia usually report gap(s) in the recollection of a particular event. The memory forgotten is usually a traumatic one, such as being raped.

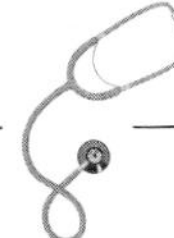

Patients suffering from dissociative amnesia can experience periods of flashbacks, nightmares, or behavioral reenactments.

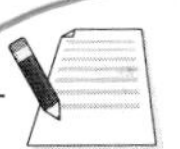

Abreaction is the strong reaction patients often get when retrieving traumatic memories.

DISSOCIATIVE FUGUE

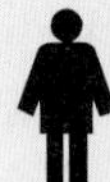

A man is found 3 days after being reported missing. He was wandering around miles away from his home and when questioned could not remember how long he had been away from home or how he got there.

Think: Dissociative fugue.

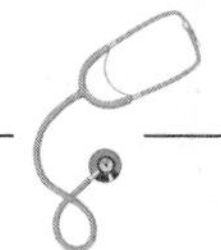

Fugue: Think about a **fug**itive who runs away and forms a new identity.

- Dissociative fugue is characterized by sudden, unexpected travel away from home, accompanied by the inability to recall one's identity or one's past.
- Patients may assume an entirely new identity and occupation after arriving in the new location.
- They are unaware of their amnesia and new identity, and they never recall the period of the fugue.
- Patients show characteristically low anxiety despite their confusion. Their affect is similar to la belle indifference of conversion responses.

DIAGNOSIS AND DSM-IV CRITERIA

- Sudden, unexpected travel away from home or work plus inability to recall one's past.
- Confusion about personal identity or assumption of new identity.
- Not due to dissociative identity disorder or the physiological effects of a substance or medical disorder.
- Symptoms cause impairment in social or occupational functioning.

EPIDEMIOLOGY

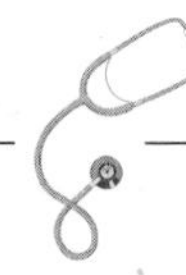

Unlike dissociative amnesia, patients with dissociative fugue are not aware that they have forgotten anything.

- Rare.
- Predisposing factors include heavy use of alcohol, major depression, history of head trauma, and epilepsy.
- Onset associated with stressful life event (dissociative fugue is often viewed as a response to a life stressor or personal conflict).

COURSE AND PROGNOSIS

The fugue usually lasts a few hours to several days but may last longer. After the episode, the patient will assume his or her old identity without ever remembering the time of the fugue.

TREATMENT

Similar to that of dissociative amnesia (see above).

DISSOCIATIVE IDENTITY DISORDER (MULTIPLE PERSONALITY DISORDER)

- A controversial diagnosis.
- Patients with dissociative identity disorder are said to have two or more distinct personalities that alternately control their behaviors and thoughts.
- Memories, habits, skills, and even physical traits (such as handedness or allergies) can be implicated. Rare studies show physiological differences (blood glucose, etc) among the personality states.

Diagnosis and DSM-IV Criteria

- Presence of two or more distinct identities.
- At least two of the identities recurrently take control of the person's behavior.
- Inability to recall personal information of one personality when the other is dominant.
- Not due to effects of substance or medical condition.

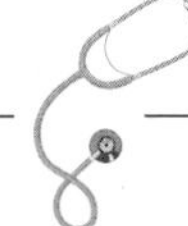

Symptoms of multiple personality disorder may be similar to those seen in borderline personality disorder, psychosis, or malingering.

Epidemiology

- Women account for up to 90% of patients.
- Most patients have experienced prior trauma, especially childhood physical or sexual abuse.
- Average age of onset is 6. The average age of diagnosis is 30.
- High incidence of comorbid major depression, anxiety disorders, borderline personality disorder, and substance abuse.
- Up to one-third of patients attempt suicide.

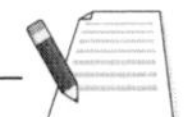

Some sources have claimed that 10 or more personality states have existed in a single patient. Other psychiatrists doubt the existence of this condition at all.

Course and Prognosis

- Course is usually chronic, with incomplete recovery.
- Worst prognosis of all dissociative disorders.
- Patients with an earlier onset have a poorer prognosis.

Treatment

- Hypnosis, drug-assisted interviewing, and insight-oriented psychotherapy.
- Pharmacotherapy as needed if comorbid disorder develops (such as major depression).

DEPERSONALIZATION DISORDER

Depersonalization disorder is characterized by persistent or recurrent feelings of detachment from one's self, environment (derealization), or social situation.

Diagnosis and DSM-IV Criteria

- Persistent or recurrent experiences of being detached from one's body or mental processes.
- Reality testing remains intact during episode.
- Causes social/occupational impairment, and cannot be accounted for by another mental or physical disorder.

Transient symptoms of depersonalization are common in normal people during times of stress.

Epidemiology

- Approximately twice as common in women than men.
- More common among adolescents and young adults.
- ↑ incidence of comorbid anxiety disorders and major depression.
- Severe stress is a predisposing factor.

Course and Prognosis

Often chronic (with either steady or intermittent course), but may remit without treatment.

Treatment

Antianxiety agents or selective serotonin reuptake inhibitors (SSRIs) to treat associated symptoms of anxiety or major depression.

DISSOCIATIVE DISORDER NOT OTHERWISE SPECIFIED

Primary dissociative disorders that share the characteristics of disruption in consciousness, memory, identity, or perception but do not meet the criteria of the other specific categories are included in this category. Many of these disorders include cultural components and are very unlikely to be seen in the wards.

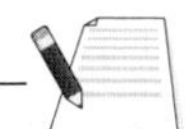

Ataque de nervios is a culturally bound trance disorder common in Puerto Rico that consists of convulsive movements, fainting, crying, and visual problems.

DSM-IV Examples

- Dissociative disorder presentations without two or more states
- Primary derealization
- Cultural-bound dissociative trance disorders
- Loss of consciousness, stupor, or coma not due to medical condition
- Ganser syndrome (the giving of approximate answers to simple questions such as how many legs do you have?)

HIGH-YIELD FACTS IN

Somatoform and Factitious Disorders

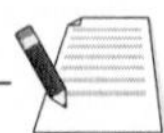

If external benefits are reached through *conscious* feigning of symptoms, this would be malingering, not secondary gain.

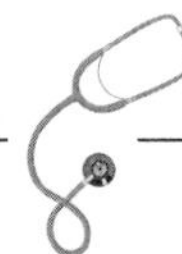

When suspecting a somatoform disorder, it is important to rule out organic causes of symptoms with a comprehensive medical workup.

Patients with somatoform disorders present with enduring physical symptoms without an identifiable organic cause, which causes significant distress or impairment in social, occupational, or other area of functioning. Although the symptoms expressed in these disorders result in primary and secondary gains, these patients truly believe that their symptoms are due to medical problems. ***They are not consciously feigning symptoms.*** Malingering, on the other hand, is when one consciously feigns symptoms in order to get something (eg, money).

- **Primary gain:** Symptoms as an unconscious defense against unacceptable *internal* conflicts (self-justification for various actions or lack of actions).
- **Secondary gain:** Symptoms that provide unconscious *external* benefits (↑ attention from others, ↓ responsibilities, avoidance of the law, etc).
- Examples of somatoform disorders include:
  - Somatization disorder
  - Conversion disorder
  - Hypochondriasis
  - Pain disorder
  - Body dysmorphic disorder
  - Undifferentiated somatoform disorder
  - Somatoform disorder not otherwise specified
- Somatoform disorders are generally more common in women. Half of patients have comorbid mental disorders, especially anxiety disorders and major depression.

Ms. Thomas is a 31-year-old woman who was referred to a psychiatrist by her gynecologist after undergoing multiple exploratory surgeries for abdominal pain and gynecologic concerns with no findings. The patient reports that she has had extensive medical problems dating back to adolescence. She reports periods of extreme abdominal pain, vomiting, diarrhea, and possible food intolerances. The obstetrician is her fourth provider because "my other doctors where not able to help me." Ms. Thomas reports fear that her current physician will also fail to relieve her distress. She was reluctant to see a psychiatrist and did so only after her obstetrician agreed to follow her after her psychiatric appointment.

Ms. Thomas states that her problems worsened in college, which was the first time she underwent surgery. She reports that due to her health problems and severe lack of energy, it took her $5^1/_2$ years to graduate from college. She did better for a year or two after college but then had a return of symptoms. She reports recently feeling very lonely and isolated because she has not been able to find a boyfriend who can tolerate her frequent illnesses. She also reports that physical intimacy is difficult for her because she finds sex painful. Additionally, she is concerned that she might lose her job due to the number of days she has missed from work due to her abdominal pain, fatigue, and weakness. On review of symptoms, she endorses periods where she is short of breath, has double vision, regular heart palpitations, irregular menses, bloating, frequent urinary tract infections and burning on urination, diffuse muscle and joint pain, frequent headaches, and periods of ringing in her ears.

What is the diagnosis?

Somatization disorder. Ms. Thomas has a history of multiple complaints in multiple organ systems, which have waxed and waned over time with no clear cause being found after extensive workup. In addition, the patient had multiple medical procedures that did not provide relief of symptoms. She also frequently changed providers.

GI complaints: diarrhea, vomiting, and bloating. Neurological complaints: double vision, ringing in ears, weakness. Reproductive system complaints: irregular menses, urinary difficulties. Pain complains: abdominal pain, pain on urination, muscle and joint pain, and headaches. These symptoms started before the age of 30, and there is a significant impairment in the patient's social and occupational functioning.

SOMATIZATION DISORDER

Patients with somatization disorder present with multiple, often nonspecific, physical symptoms involving many organ systems. They seek treatment from many doctors, often resulting in extensive lab work, diagnostic procedures, hospitalizations, and/or surgeries.

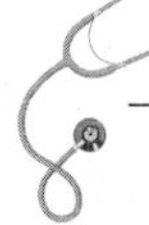

Five to ten percent of patients presenting in primary care have a somatization disorder.

DIAGNOSIS AND DSM-IV CRITERIA

- Onset **before age 30.**
- At least four pain symptoms.
- At least two gastrointestinal (GI) symptoms.
- At least one sexual or reproductive symptom.
- At least one pseudoneurological symptom, not limited to pain.
- Cannot be explained by a general medical condition or substance use.
- When a general medical condition is present, physical complaints are in excess of what would be expected.
- Symptoms must not be intentionally produced.

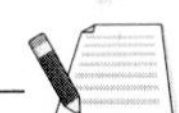

Somatization disorder patients typically express lots of concern over their condition and chronically perseverate over this, whereas conversion disorder patients often have an abrupt onset of their "disability" (blindness, etc) and the patient usually appears apathetic.

EPIDEMIOLOGY

- Incidence in females 5–20 times that of males.
- Lifetime prevalence: 0.1–0.5%.
- Fifty percent have comorbid medical disorder.
- Thirty percent concordance in identical twins.
- Patients frequently report history of sexual and/or physical abuse.

TREATMENT AND PROGNOSIS

- The course is usually chronic and debilitating. Symptoms may periodically improve and then worsen under stress.
- The patient should have regularly scheduled visits with a single primary care physician, who limits, but does not eliminate, medical workups.
- Address psychological issues slowly. Patients will likely resist referral to a mental health professional.

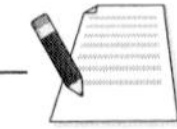

Somatization—**So many** physical complaints.

CONVERSION DISORDER

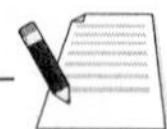

Conversion disorder: Patients **convert** psychiatric problems to a neurological problem and then spontaneously **convert** back to normal.

- Patients with conversion disorder have at least one neurological symptom (sensory or motor) that cannot be explained by a medical disorder.
- Onset is usually preceded or exacerbated by a psychological stressor, although the patient may not connect the two.
- Patients are often surprisingly calm and unconcerned *(la belle indifference)* when describing their symptoms.
- Examples of neurological symptoms include blindness, paralysis, paresthesia.

Diagnosis and DSM-IV Criteria

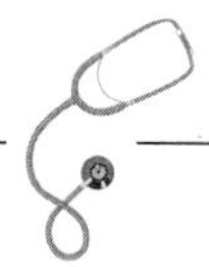

Conversion-like presentations in elderly patients have a higher likelihood of representing a real neurological deficit.

- At least one neurological symptom.
- Psychological factors associated with initiation or exacerbation of symptoms.
- Not intentionally feigned or produced.
- Cannot be explained by medical condition or substance use.
- Causes significant distress or impairment in social or occupational functioning or warrants medical evaluation.
- Not limited to pain or sexual dysfunction, and not better accounted for by a different mental disorder.
- **Common symptoms:** Shifting paralysis, blindness, mutism, paresthesias, seizures, globus hystericus (sensation of lump in throat).

Epidemiology

- More common in women than men
- Onset at any age, but most often in adolescence or early adulthood
- High incidence of comorbid schizophrenia, major depression, or anxiety disorders

Treatment and Prognosis

- Treatments may include insight-oriented psychotherapy, hypnosis, or relaxation therapy if needed. Most patients spontaneously recover.
- Symptoms may be brief or last for several weeks or longer. Twenty-five percent will eventually have future episodes, especially during times of stress.

HYPOCHONDRIASIS

Diagnosis and DSM-IV Criteria

- Preoccupation with fear of having or contracting a serious disease, based on misinterpreting bodily symptoms
- Persists despite medical evaluation and reassurance
- Not of delusional intensity and not restricted to a circumscribed concern about appearance
- Significant impairment in functioning
- Persists for at least **6 months**
- Not better accounted for by another mental disorder

EPIDEMIOLOGY

- Men are affected as often as women.
- Average age of onset: 20–30.
- Eighty percent have coexisting major depression or anxiety disorder.

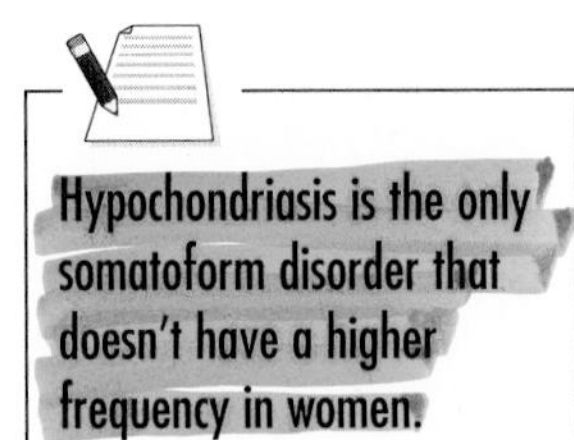

Hypochondriasis is the only somatoform disorder that doesn't have a higher frequency in women.

TREATMENT

- Regularly scheduled visits to one primary care physician.
- Comorbid anxiety and depression should be treated with selective serotonin reuptake inhibitors (SSRIs) or other psychotropic medications.
- Cognitive-behavioral therapy (CBT) seems to be most useful of psychotherapies.

PROGNOSIS

- Episodic—symptoms may wax and wane periodically.
- Exacerbations occur commonly under stress.
- Up to 50% of patients improve significantly.
- Better prognostic factors include higher socioeconomic status, treatment-responsive anxiety or depression, and absence of comorbid medical conditions and personality disorders.

BODY DYSMORPHIC DISORDER

- Patients with body dysmorphic disorder are preoccupied with body parts that they perceive as flawed or defective, having strong beliefs that they are unattractive or repulsive.
- Though their physical imperfections are either minimal or completely imagined, patients view them as severe and grotesque.
- They are very self-conscious about their appearance.
- They spend significant time trying to correct perceived flaws with makeup, dermatological procedures, or plastic surgery.

DIAGNOSIS AND DSM-IV CRITERIA

- Preoccupation with an imagined defect in appearance or excessive concern about a slight physical anomaly
- Must cause significant distress in the patient's life
- Not better accounted for by another mental disorder

EPIDEMIOLOGY

- More common in women than men
- More common in unmarried than married persons
- Average age of onset: Between 15 and 20
- High comorbidity with depression, anxiety disorders, and psychotic disorders

TREATMENT AND PROGNOSIS

- Surgical or dermatological procedures are routinely unsuccessful in pleasing the patient.
- SSRIs may reduce symptoms in 50% of patients.
- The onset is usually gradual. Symptoms may be chronic, or they may wax and wane in intensity.

PAIN DISORDER

- Patients with pain disorder have prolonged, severe discomfort without an adequate medical explanation.
- The pain often coexists with a medical condition but is not directly caused by it or not *fully* accounted for by it.
- Patients often have a history of multiple visits to doctors. Pain disorder can be acute (< 6 months) or chronic (> 6 months).

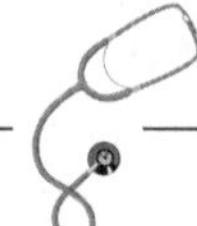

Patients with pain disorder may have a real medical condition (multiple sclerosis, back injury, etc) but with pain symptoms that are far in excess of the disease pathology.

Diagnosis and DSM-IV Criteria

- Patient's main complaint is pain at one or more anatomic sites, of sufficient severity to warrant clinical attention.
- The pain causes significant distress or impairment in the patient's life.
- Psychological factors play an important role in the pain.
- Not intentionally produced.
- Not better accounted for by a mental disorder or meet criteria for dyspareunia.

Epidemiology

- Women are two times as likely as men to have pain disorder.
- Average age of onset: 30–50.
- ↑ incidence in first-degree relatives.
- ↑ incidence in blue-collar workers.
- Patients have higher incidence of major depression, anxiety disorders, and substance abuse.

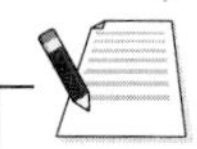

Major depression can exacerbate the symptoms of pain disorder.

Treatment and Prognosis

- Treatment includes SSRIs, biofeedback, hypnosis, and psychotherapy.
- Analgesics are not helpful, and patients often become dependent on them.
- Pain disorder usually ↑ in intensity for the first several months and often becomes chronic and disabling.

FACTITIOUS DISORDER

- Patients with factitious disorder intentionally produce medical or psychological symptoms in order to assume the role of a sick patient.
- They often do this in a way that can cause real danger (central line infections, insulin injections, etc).
- *Primary gain* is a prominent feature of this disorder.

Diagnosis and DSM-IV Criteria

- Patients **intentionally** produce signs of physical or mental disorders.
- They produce the symptoms to assume the sick role *(primary gain).*
- Lack of secondary gain distinguishes factitious disorder from malingering.
- There are no external incentives (such as monetary reward, etc) as in malingering.
- Intentional, conscious production of physical or psychological signs and symptoms.

- **Commonly feigned symptoms:**
  - *Psychiatric*—hallucinations, depression, pseudologia fantastica
  - *Medical*—fever (by heating the thermometer), abdominal pain, seizures, skin lesions, and hematuria

EPIDEMIOLOGY

- Can be present in as high as 5% of hospitalized patients.
- Higher incidence in hospital and health care workers (who have learned how to feign symptoms).
- Associated with higher intelligence, poor sense of identity, and poor sexual adjustment.
- Many patients have a history of child abuse or neglect.

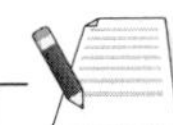

Münchhausen syndrome is another name for factitious disorder with predominantly physical complaints. **Münchhausen syndrome by proxy** is intentionally producing symptoms in someone else who is under one's care (usually one's children).

TREATMENT AND PROGNOSIS

- Collect collateral information from medical treaters and family. Collaborate with primary care physician to avoid unnecessary procedures.
- Avoid early confrontation. Patients who are confronted while in the hospital often leave against medical advice and seek hospitalization elsewhere.
- Repeated and long-term hospitalizations are common.

MALINGERING

A patient claims that he has frequent episodes of "seizures," starts on medications, and joins an epilepsy support group. It becomes known that he is doing this in order to collect disability money. *Diagnosis?* **Malingering.** In contrast, in **factitious disorder,** patients look for some kind of emotional gain by playing the "sick role," such as sympathy from the physician. The fundamental difference between malingering and factitious disorder is in the intention of the patient; in malingering, the motivation is external, whereas in factitious disorder, the motivation is internal.

- Malingering involves the feigning of physical or psychological symptoms in order to achieve personal gain.
- Common external motivations include avoiding the police, receiving room and board, obtaining narcotics, and receiving monetary compensation.

PRESENTATION

- Patients usually present with multiple vague complaints that do not conform to a known medical condition.
- They often have a long medical history with many hospital stays.
- They are generally uncooperative and refuse to accept a good prognosis even after extensive medical evaluation.
- Their symptoms improve once their desired objective is obtained.

EPIDEMIOLOGY

- Common in hospitalized patients
- More common in men than women

REVIEW OF DISTINGUISHING FEATURES

- **Somatoform disorders:** Patients *believe* they are ill and do not intentionally produce or feign symptoms.
- **Factitious disorders:** Patients intentionally produce symptoms of real illness because of a desire to assume the *sick role,* not for external rewards.
- **Malingering:** Patients intentionally produce or feign symptoms for *external rewards.*

HIGH-YIELD FACTS IN

Impulse Control Disorders

Impulse control disorders are characterized by a predisposed inability to resist unplanned, rapid reactions toward internal or external stimuli without regard for negative consequences, that may cause harm to oneself or to others. Impulse control disorders are not caused by another mental condition, medical condition, or substance use.

Core qualities of the impulse control disorders are as follows:

1. Repetitive or compulsive engagement in behavior despite adverse consequences
2. Little control over the negative behavior
3. Anxiety or craving experienced prior to engagement in impulsive behavior
4. Relief or satisfaction during or after completion of the behavior

Mr. Baker is a 27-year-old married accountant who arrives at the outpatient psychiatry clinic complaining of difficulty in managing his anger. He has no prior psychiatric history, but reports that he has had difficulty controlling his temper since adolescence. He reports that he is easily angered by small occurrences, such as his wife's failing to make coffee or a coworker's forgetting a pen at work. He reacts quickly and in a volatile way, describing it as "going from 0 to 60 before I know it." Mr. Baker feels that he is unable to control his anger, has thrown objects in fits of rage, and has made threatening statements to his wife and coworkers in the past. One coworker has recently threatened to pursue legal action.

Mr. Baker describes these episodes as brief, lasting only 10–15 minutes, and feeling embarrassed shortly after the episode has transpired. He is concerned he may lose his job because of his behavior, and he worries about the fate of his relationships. The patient denies any history of drug or alcohol abuse.

What is his most likely diagnosis?

Based on Mr. Baker's history, his most likely diagnosis is intermittent explosive disorder. However, it is important to recognize that impulsivity is a common characteristic of other Axis I and Axis II diagnoses, and these must be ruled out prior to diagnosing a patient with this disorder.

What would be your recommended treatment?

Treatment for this disorder usually involves the use of medications used to treat impulsive aggression. These include selective serotonin reuptake inhibitors (SSRIs), fluoxetine in particular; anticonvulsants; lithium (mood stabilizer); antipsychotics; and propranolol. Individual psychotherapy is difficult and ineffective given the nature of the disease and lack of individual control. However, imaginal exposure therapy, relaxation training, and dialectical behavioral therapy have been effectively used in the treatment of anger management. Group therapy and/or family therapy may be useful to create behavior plans to help manage episodes.

What are associated laboratory findings?

Aside from low mean 5-hydroxyindoleacetic acid (5-HIAA) concentration that have been found in the cerebrospinal fluid of some impulsive individuals, there may also be nonspecific electroencephalographic findings or abnormalities on neuropsychological testing.

INTERMITTENT EXPLOSIVE DISORDER

DIAGNOSIS AND DSM-IV CRITERIA

- Recurrent outbursts of aggression that result in assault against people or property.
- Outbursts and aggression are out of proportion to the triggering event or stressor.
- Aggression is not better explained by another psychiatric diagnosis.
- Each episode of explosive behavior often remits quickly and spontaneously, often leaving patients feeling remorseful and distressed.

EPIDEMIOLOGY/ETIOLOGY

- More common in men than women.
- Onset usually in late teens and may progress in severity until middle age.
- Genetic, perinatal, environmental, and neurobiological factors may play a role in etiology. Patients may have history of child abuse, head trauma, or seizures.

> Low levels of serotonin have been shown to be associated with impulsiveness and aggression.

TREATMENT

- Treatment involves use of selective serotonin reuptake inhibitors (SSRIs), anticonvulsants, lithium (mood stabilizer), and propranolol.
- Individual psychotherapy is difficult and ineffective given the nature of the disease and lack of individual control.
- Group therapy and/or family therapy may be useful to create behavior plans to help manage episodes.

KLEPTOMANIA

DIAGNOSIS AND DSM-IV CRITERIA

- Inability to resist uncontrollable urges to steal objects that are not needed for personal use or monetary reasons.
- Pleasure or relief is experienced while stealing; however, intense guilt and shame are often reported by those with the disorder.
- Objects stolen are typically given or thrown away, returned, or hoarded.

EPIDEMIOLOGY/ETIOLOGY

- More common in women than men, though severity of symptoms are not gender biased.
- Symptoms often occur during times of stress.
- Occurs in under 5% of shoplifters.
- ↑ incidence of comorbid mood disorders, eating disorders, and obsessive-compulsive disorder (OCD).
- Biological factors and family dysfunction in childhood may contribute to etiology.
- Course of illness is usually chronic.

> One-fourth of patients with bulimia nervosa have comorbid kleptomania.

TREATMENT

Treatment may include insight-oriented psychotherapy, behavior therapy such as systematic desensitization and aversive conditioning, and SSRIs. There is some anecdotal evidence for naltrexone use.

PATHOLOGICAL GAMBLING

DIAGNOSIS AND DSM-IV CRITERIA

Persistent and recurrent maladaptive gambling behavior, as evidenced by five or more of the following:

1. Preoccupation with gambling
2. Need to gamble with increasing amount of money to achieve pleasure
3. Repeated and unsuccessful attempts to cut down on gambling
4. Restlessness or irritability when attempting to stop gambling
5. Gambling done to escape problems or relieve dysphoria
6. Returning to reclaim losses after gambling
7. Lying to therapist or family members to hide level of gambling
8. Committing illegal acts to finance gambling
9. Jeopardizing relationships or job because of gambling
10. Relying on others to financially support gambling

EPIDEMIOLOGY/ETIOLOGY

- Prevalence: 1–3% of adults in the United States.
- Men represent approximately two-thirds of cases.
- High rates in adolescents and young adults, lower rates in older adults, marked by periods of abstinence and relapse.
- ↑ incidence of mood disorders, anxiety disorders, and OCD.
- Predisposing factors include loss of a parent during childhood, inappropriate parental discipline during childhood, attention deficit/hyperactivity disorder, and lack of family emphasis on budgeting or saving money.
- Etiology may involve genetic, biological, environmental, and neurochemical factors.
- One-third will achieve recovery without treatment.

TREATMENT

- Participation in Gamblers Anonymous (a 12-step program) is the most effective treatment.
- After 3 months of abstinence from gambling, insight-oriented psychotherapy may be attempted.
- Important to treat comorbid mood disorders, anxiety disorders, and substance abuse problems with SSRIs, mood stabilizers, or opioid antagonists.

TRICHOTILLOMANIA

DIAGNOSIS AND DSM-IV CRITERIA

- Recurrent, repetitive, intentional pulling out of one's hair causing visible hair loss.
- Usually involves the scalp, though can include eyebrows, eyelashes, and facial and pubic hair.
- Tension is experienced immediately before the pulling behavior, and pleasure or relief occurs afterwards.
- Causes significant distress or impairment in daily functioning.

EPIDEMIOLOGY/ETIOLOGY

- Seen in 1–3% of the population.
- More common in women than in men.
- Onset usually during childhood or adolescence, and is associated with a stressful event in 25% of patients.
- It is thought that the texture of the hair acts as a trigger for behavior.
- Commonly causes significant occupational and social dysfunction.
- Etiology may involve biological, genetic, and environmental factors, such as problems in relationship with parent, recent loss of an important object or figure, etc.
- ↑ incidence of comorbid OCD, obsessive-compulsive personality disorder (OCPD), mood disorders, and borderline personality disorder.
- Course may be chronic or remitting; adult onset is generally more difficult to treat.

TREATMENT

- Treatment includes medications such as SSRIs, antipsychotics, or lithium.
- Behavioral interventions such as hypnosis, relaxation techniques, substituting another behavior, or positive reinforcement may have some therapeutic benefit.

PYROMANIA

DIAGNOSIS AND DSM-IV CRITERIA

- At least one episode of deliberate fire setting.
- Tension or arousal experienced before the act, and pleasure, gratification, or relief experienced when setting fires and subsequent consequences.
- Fascination with, interest in, curiosity about, or attraction to fire and consequences.
- Purpose of fire setting is not for monetary gain, expression of anger, or making a political statement, and is not due to a hallucination or delusion.

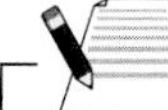

Pyromania is the impulse to start fires to relieve tension, typically with feelings of gratification or relief afterward.

EPIDEMIOLOGY/ETIOLOGY

- Long thought to primarily affect men; however, research suggests the ratio may be equal in men and women.
- Mean age of onset is late adolescence.
- Prognosis is better in children than adults; with treatment, children often recover completely.
- Course can be chronic if untreated.

TREATMENT

Treatment involves use of behavior therapy, supervision, and SSRIs.

NOTES

HIGH-YIELD FACTS IN

Eating Disorders

DEFINITION

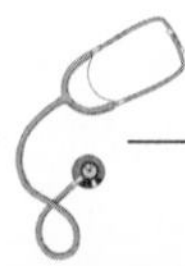

Suspect an eating disorder? Ask the patient what is the most/least she has weighed, her ideal body weight, if she counts calories/fat/carbs/protein, how much she exercises, if she binges and purges, and if she has food rituals (eg, drinking water between bites).

Eating disorders include anorexia nervosa and bulimia nervosa. Patients with anorexia or bulimia have a disturbed body image and use extensive measures to avoid gaining weight (vomiting, laxatives, diuretics, enemas, fasting, and excessive exercise). Binge-eating disorder is listed under the *Diagnostic and Statistical Manual of Mental Disorders*, 4th ed., Text Revision (DSM-IV-TR) category of Eating Disorder NOS (not otherwise specified).

Ms. Williams is a 17-year-old Caucasian woman without prior psychiatric history who is brought to the emergency room by ambulance after her parents called 911 when they found her having a seizure in their living room. She was admitted to the medical intensive care unit in status epilepticus and was quickly stabilized with intramuscular lorazepam and fosphenytoin loading. Her height is 5 feet 6 inches, she is of medium build, and her weight is 101 pounds (BMI 16.3 kg/m^2). She does not suffer any medical conditions, and this is her first seizure. Laboratory workup shows an electrolyte imbalance as the most likely cause for her seizures. Although initially reluctant, she admits to purging with the use of ipecac several times this week. She reports that although she normally restricts her daily caloric intake to 500 calories, she regularly induces vomiting if her weight is above 100 pounds. Her last menstrual cycle was 1 year ago. Psychiatric consultation is requested in order to confirm her diagnosis.

As the psychiatrist on call, you evaluate Ms. Williams and find that she appears underweight and younger than her stated age. She is in mild distress, has a nastrogastic tube in place, and exhibits poor eye contact. She reports feeling "sad" and admitted to experiencing constant preoccupation about her physical appearance and says, "I'm fat; I hate my body." She also reports insomnia, low energy levels, and a history of self-harm behavior by cutting her forearms. She reports that she is careful in hiding her symptoms from her parents, whom she describes as strict disciplinarians. She also expresses concerns that she will disappoint them.

Ms. Williams's parents describe her as a perfectionist. They say that she is involved in multiple school activities, takes advanced placement classes, and has been recently concerned about being accepted at her college of choice. They report that she has maintained a 4.0 grade point average in high school, and they expect her to become a doctor. Her parents have noticed that she is underweight and rarely see her eat, but have attributed this to stress from her many academic pursuits. Ms. Williams's mother receives treatment for obsessive-compulsive disorder.

What is Ms. Williams's most likely diagnosis?

The most likely diagnosis is anorexia nervosa—binge-eating/purging type. As described above, she refuses to weigh more than 100 pounds, which is significantly below the minimal normal weight for her height. Despite being underweight, she expresses intense fear of gaining weight, has a disturbance in the way her body shape is experienced, and has missed her menstrual period for more than three cycles. In addition, she has engaged in binge-eating/purging behavior regularly. You should also explore for comorbid depression, anxiety, and personality disorder. Remember that malnutrition in itself can → some of the symptoms experienced in depression and that many patients show an improvement in their mood when nutrition is replenished.

What are some of the medical complications associated with this condition?

Patients with anorexia nervosa might present with bradycardia, ortostatic hypotension, arrhythmias, QTc prolongation, and ST-T wave changes in electrocardiogram, as well as anemia and leukopenia. They might also experience cognitive impairment, evidence of enlarged ventricles and/or ↓ gray and white matter on brain imaging, and peripheral neuropathy. Lanugo and muscle wasting sometimes become evident. Aside from amenorrhea, loss of libido is commonly reported. In patients who regularly engage in self-induced vomiting, parotid enlargement, ↑ amylase levels, and electrolyte imbalances (eg, hypokalemia) commonly occur as a result.

ANOREXIA NERVOSA

Patients with anorexia nervosa are preoccupied with their weight, their body image, and being thin. There are two main subdivisions:

- **Restrictive type:** Has not regularly engaged in binge-eating or purging behavior; often with obsessive-compulsive personality traits
- **Binge-eating/purging type:** Eat in binges followed by self-induced vomiting, using laxatives, excessively exercising, and/or using diuretics

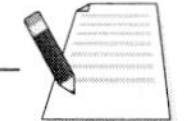

Both anorexia and bulimia are characterized for a desire for thinness. Both may binge and purge. Anorexia nervosa involves **low body weight,** and this distinguishes it from bulimia.

DIAGNOSIS AND DSM-IV CRITERIA

- Refusal to maintain a minimally normal body weight for one's age and height (< 85% of ideal body weight or body mass index [BMI] < 17.5 kg/m^2)
- Intense fear of gaining weight or becoming fat
- Disturbed body image, undue influence of weight or shape on self-evaluation, or denial of the seriousness of the current low body weight
- Amenorrhea in postmenarchal females (ie, absence of at least three consecutive menstrual cycles)

PHYSICAL FINDINGS AND MEDICAL COMPLICATIONS

- The medical complications of eating disorders are related to weight loss and purging (vomiting and laxative abuse).
- Physical manifestations: Amenorrhea, cold intolerance/hypothermia, hypotension (especially orthostasis), braydcardia, arrhythmia, acute coronary syndrome, cardiomyopathy, mitral valve prolapse, constipation, lanugo hair, alopecia, edema, dehydration, peripheral neuropathy, seizures, hypothyrodism, osteopenia, osteoporosis.
- Laboratory/imaging abnormalities: Hyponatremia, hypochloremic hypokalemic alkalosis (if vomiting), arrhythmia (especially QTc prolongation), hypercholesterolemia, transaminitis, leuokopenia, anemia (normocytic normochromic), elevated blood urea nitrogen (BUN), ↑ growth hormone (GH), ↑ cortisol, reduced gonadotropins (luteinizing hormone [LH], follicle-stimulating hormone [FSH]), reduced sex steroid hormones (estrogen, testosterone), hypothyrpoidism, hypoglycemia, osteopenia.

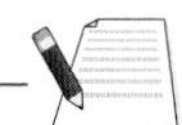

Classic example of anorexia nervosa: An extremely thin amenorrheic teenage girl whose mother says she eats very little does aerobics for 2 hours a day and *ritualistically* does 400 sit-ups every day (500 if she has "overeaten").

EPIDEMIOLOGY

- Ninety to ninety-five percent are women.
- Lifetime prevalence: 1%.
- Bimodal age of onset (age 13–14: hormonal influences; age 17–18: environmental influences).
- More common in industrialized countries where food is abundant and a thin body ideal is held.
- Common in sports that involve thinness, revealing attire, subjective judging, and weight classes (eg, running, ballet, wrestling, diving, cheerleading, figure skating).

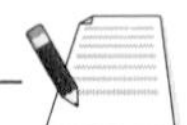

> Anorexia Versus Major Depressive Disorder
> *Anorexia nervosa:* Patients have ***good appetite*** but starve themselves due to distorted body image. They are often quite preoccupied with food, preparing it for others, etc, but do not eat it themselves.
> *Major depressive disorder:* Patients usually have *poor appetite,* which → weight loss. These patients have no interest in food.

ETIOLOGY

- Multifactorial.
- Genetics: Higher concordance in monozygotic than dizygotic twin studies.
- Psychodynamic theories: Difficulty with separation and autonomy (eg, parental enmeshment) and struggle to gain control, attempt to halt or reverse secondary sexual characteristics.
- Social theories: Exaggeration of social values (achievement, control, and perfectionism), idealization of thin body and prepubescent appearance in Western world, ↑ prevalence of dieting at earlier ages.

DIFFERENTIAL DIAGNOSIS

- Medical conditions: Endocrine disorders (eg, hypothalamic disease, diabetes mellitus, hyperthyroidism), gastrointestinal illnesses (eg, malabsorption, inflammatory bowel disease), genetic disorders (eg, Turner syndrome, Gaucher disease), cancer, AIDS.
- Psychiatric disorders: Major depression, bulimia, or other mental disorder (such as somatization disorder or schizophrenia).

> **Refeeding syndrome** occurs when severely malnourished patients are refed too quickly. Look for fluid retention and ↓ levels of phosphorus, magnesium, and calcium. Complications include arrhythmias, respiratory failure, delirium, and seizures. Replace electrolytes and slow the feedings.

COURSE AND PROGNOSIS

- Chronic and relapsing illness. Variable course—may completely recover, have fluctuating symptoms with relapses, or progressively deteriorate.
- Mortality rate is cumulative, and approximately 10% due to starvation, **suicide,** or cardiac failure. Rates of suicide are approximately 57 times higher than normal.

TREATMENT

- Food is the best medicine!
- Patients may be treated as outpatients unless they are more than 20% below ideal body weight or if there are serious medical or psychiatric complications, in which case they should be hospitalized for supervised refeeding.
- Treatment involves behavioral therapy, family therapy (eg, Maudsley approach), and supervised weight-gain programs.
- Selective serotonin reuptake inhibitors (SSRIs) have not been effective in the treatment of anorexia nervosa, which is believed to be due to inadequate dietary intake of tryptophan, the precursor of serotonin.

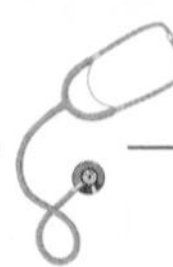

> When a patient with anorexia learns that weight gain is a common side effect, she may refuse medication.

Birth defects - prior eating disorders:
- prematurity
- small for gestational age
- miscarriage
- postpartum depression

osteoporosis

- Low-dose second-generation antipsychotics may treat excessive preoccupation with weight and food in addition to independently promoting weight gain.
- Benzodiazepines may also be administered prior to meals to reduce preprandial anxiety.

BULIMIA NERVOSA

Bulimia nervosa involves binge eating combined with behaviors intended to counteract weight gain, such as vomiting; use of laxatives, enemas, or diuretics; or excessive exercise. Patients are embarrassed by their binge eating and are overly concerned with body weight. However, unlike patients with anorexia, they usually maintain a normal weight (and may be overweight). There are two subcategories of bulimia:

- **Purging type:** Involves vomiting, laxatives, enemas, or diuretics
- **Nonpurging type:** Involves excessive exercise or fasting

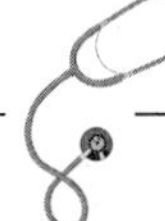

Unlike patients with anorexia nervosa, bulimic patients usually maintain a **normal weight,** and their symptoms are more **ego-dystonic** (distressing); they are therefore more likely to seek help.

DIAGNOSIS AND DSM-IV CRITERIA

- Recurrent episodes of binge eating.
- Recurrent, inappropriate attempts to compensate for overeating and prevent weight gain (such as laxative abuse, vomiting, diuretics, or excessive exercise).
- The binge eating and compensatory behaviors occur at least twice a week for 3 months.
- Perception of self-worth is excessively influenced by body weight and shape.

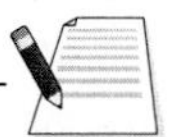

Binge eating is defined by excessive food intake within a 2-hour period accompanied by a sense of lack of control.

PHYSICAL FINDINGS AND MEDICAL COMPLICATIONS

- Patients with anorexia and bulimia may have similar medical complications related to weight loss and vomiting.
- Physical manifestations: Salivary gland enlargement (sialadenosis), dental erosion/caries, callouses/abrasions on dorsum of hand ("Russell's sign" from self-induced vomiting), petechieae, peripheral edema, aspiration.
- Laboratory/imaging abnormalities: Hypochloremic hypokalemic alkalosis, metabolic acidosis (laxative abuse), elevated bicarbonate (compensation), hypernatremia, ↑ BUN, ↑ amylase, altered thryroid hormone and cortisol homeostasis, esophagitis.

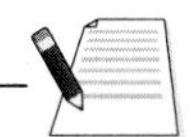

Cortisol is often ↑ in patients with anorexia nervosa.

EPIDEMIOLOGY

- Lifetime prevalence: 1–4%.
- Significantly more common in women (90–95%) than men.
- Onset is in late adolescence or early adulthood.
- More common in developed countries.
- High incidence of comorbid mood disorders, anxiety disorders, impulse control disorders, substance abuse, sexual abuse, and ↑ prevalence of cluster B and C personality disorders.

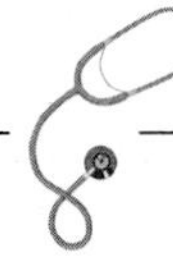

Recurrent episodes of binge eating is the most diagnostic feature of bulimia nervosa, according to DSM-IV.

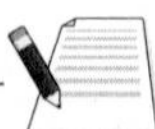

Anorexia nervosa and bulimia nervosa are risk factors for developing cardiac arrhythmias due to electrolyte disturbances such as hypokalemia.

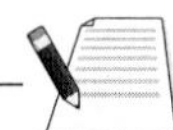

Fluoxetine is an effective medication for bulimia.

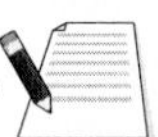

Classic example of bulimia nervosa: A 20-year-old college student is referred by her dentist because of multiple dental caries. She is normal weight for her height but feels that "she needs to lose 15 pounds." She reluctantly admits to eating a large quantity of food in a short period of time and then inducing gagging.

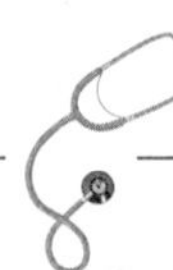

In patients with bulimia, make sure to check that they aren't on medications that could further lower their seizure threshold, such as the antidepressant Wellbutrin (buproprion).

Etiology

- Multifactorial, with similar factors as for anorexia (eg, genetics and social theories)
- Psychodynamic theories: Masochistic displays of control and displaced anger over one's body

Course and Prognosis

- Chronic and relapsing illness.
- Better prognosis than anorexia nervosa.
- Symptoms are usually exacerbated by stressful conditions.
- One-half recover fully with treatment; one-half have chronic course with fluctuating symptoms.

Treatment

- Antidepressants plus therapy (more effective combo for bulimia than for anorexia).
- SSRIs are first-line medication.
- Fluoxetine is the only FDA-approved medication for bulimia (60–80 mg/day).
- Often requires multiple medications.
- Therapy includes cognitive-behavioral therapy, interpersonal psychotherapy, group therapy, and family therapy.
- Avoid buproprion due to its potential side effect to lower seizure threshold.

BINGE-EATING DISORDER

Binge-eating disorder falls under the DSM-IV-TR category of Eating Disorder NOS. Patients with this disorder suffer emotional distress over their binge eating, but they do not try to control their weight by purging or restricting calories, as do anorexics or bulimics. Unlike anorexia and bulimia, patients with binge-eating disorder are not fixated on their body shape and weight.

Diagnosis and DSM-IV-TR Research Criteria

- Recurrent episodes of binge eating (eating an excessive amount of food in a 2-hour period associated with a lack of control).
- Severe distress over binge eating.
- Binge eating occurs at least 2 days a week for 6 months and is not associated with compensatory behaviors (such as vomiting, laxative use, etc).
- Three or more of the following are present:
  1. Eating very rapidly
  2. Eating until uncomfortably full
  3. Eating large amounts when not hungry
  4. Eating alone due to embarrassment over eating habits
  5. Feeling disgusted, depressed, or guilty after overeating

Treatment

- Treatment involves individual psychotherapy and behavioral therapy with a strict diet and exercise program. Comorbid mood disorders or anxiety disorders should be treated as necessary.
- Pharmacotherapy may be used adjunctively to promote weight loss, including:
  - Stimulants (such as phentermine and amphetamine)—suppress appetite.
  - Orlistat (Xenical)—inhibits pancreatic lipase, thus decreasing amount of fat absorbed from gastrointestinal tract.
  - Sibutramine (Meridia)—inhibits reuptake of norepinephrine, serotonin, and dopamine.

Sleep disorders affect as many as 50–70 million people in the United States. Current data demonstrate a high rate of comorbidity between sleep disorders and various psychiatric illnesses. Disturbances in sleep can potentiate and/or exacerbate psychological distress.

NORMAL SLEEP-WAKE CYCLE

- Normal sleep-wake cycle is defined in terms of characteristic changes in several physiological parameters, including brain wave activity, eye movements, and motor activity.
- The two stages of normal sleep are rapid eye movement (REM) sleep and non–rapid eye movement (NREM) sleep.
- About every 90 minutes, NREM sleep alternates with REM sleep.
- NREM induces transition from the waking state to deep sleep.
- Progression through NREM sleep results in slower brain wave patterns and higher arousal thresholds.
- In REM sleep, brain wave patterns resemble the electroencephalogram (EEG) of an aroused person.
- Awakening from REM sleep is associated with vivid dream recall.

SLEEP DISORDERS

- Classified as either:
  - **Dyssomnias:** Insufficient, excessive, or altered timing of sleep
  - **Parasomnias:** Unusual sleep-related behaviors
- When taking a sleep history, ask about:
  - Activities prior to bedtime that may interfere with restful sleep
  - Bed partner history
  - Consequence on waking function; quality of life
  - Drug regimen, medications
  - Exacerbating or relieving factors
  - Frequency and duration
  - Genetic factors or family history
  - Habits (alcohol consumption, use of caffeine, nicotine, illicit substances, and hypnotics)

DYSSOMNIAS

Dyssomnias are disorders that make it difficult to fall or remain asleep (insomnias), or of excessive daytime sleepiness (hypersomnias).

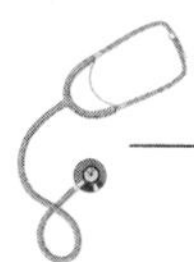

Breathing-related disorders are the most common of the hypersomnias and include obstructive sleep apnea and central sleep apnea.

Primary Insomnia

- Refers to number of symptoms that interfere with duration and/or quality of sleep despite adequate opportunity for sleep. Symptoms may include:
  - Difficulty initiating sleep **(sleep-onset insomnia)**
  - Frequent nocturnal awakenings **(middle-of-the night or sleep-maintenance insomnia)**

- Early morning awakenings **(late night or sleep-offset insomnia)**
- Waking up feeling fatigued and unrefreshed **(nonrestorative sleep)**
- **Acute insomnia** (between 1 and 4 weeks) is generally associated with stress or changes in sleep schedule and usually resolves spontaneously.
- **Chronic insomnia** lasts ≥ 1 month to years and is associated with reduced quality of life and ↑ risk of psychiatric illness.

DSM-IV Criteria

- Difficulty initiating or maintaining sleep, or nonrestorative sleep, for at least 1 month
- Causes clinically significant distress or impairment in functioning
- Does not occur exclusively in the course of another sleep disorder
- Does not occur exclusively in the course of another mental disorder
- Not due to a substance or general medical condition

Epidemiology

Prevalence: 5–10%.

Etiology

- Subclinical mood and/or anxiety disorders
- Preoccupation with a perceived inability to sleep
- Bedtime behavior not conducive to adequate sleep **(poor sleep hygiene)**
- Idiopathic

Treatment

- Sleep hygiene measures
- Cognitive-behavioral therapy (CBT)
- Pharmacotherapy:
  - Benzodiazepines:
    - Reduce sleep latency and nocturnal awakening.
    - As effective as CBT during short periods of treatment (4–8 weeks); insufficient evidence to support long-term efficacy.
    - Side effects include development of tolerance, addiction, daytime sleepiness, and rebound insomnia.
    - In the elderly, falls, confusion, and dizziness are of particular concern.
  - Non-benzodiazepines:
    - Includes zolpidem (Ambien), eszopiclone (Lunesta) and zaleplon (Sonata).
    - Effective for short-term treatment.
    - Associated with low incidence of daytime sleepiness and orthostatic hypotension.
    - In the elderly, zolpidem causes an ↑ risk of falls and may induce cognitive impairment.
  - Antidepressants:
    - Trazodone, amitriptyline, and doxepin (off-label use).
    - Side effects include sedation, dizziness, and psychomotor impairment.
    - Trazodone is the most prescribed sedating antidepressant for patients with chronic insomnia and depressive symptoms.

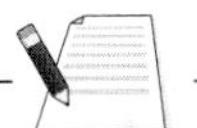

CBT is considered first-line therapy for chronic insomnia.

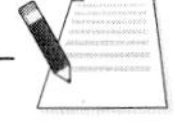

Insomnia is the most common approved and accepted reason to put a patient on long-term benzodiazepines.

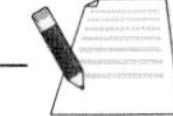

REM sleep is characterized by an ↑ in blood pressure, heart rate, and respiratory rate.

Obstructive Sleep Apnea

A 40-year-old businessman states that over the past 2 years, he has had trouble staying awake for more than 2 hours before falling asleep. He has a hard time sleeping through the night. Meanwhile, his performance at work is suffering. *Diagnosis?* This could be many things, but you must always consider obstructive sleep apnea in addition to primary insomnia, narcolepsy, etc.

Chronic breathing-related disorder characterized by repetitive collapse of the upper airway usually associated with a reduction in blood oxygen saturation.

Features

- Excessive daytime sleepiness
- Apneic episodes characterized by cessation of breathing
- Sleep fragmentation (sleep maintenance insomnia)
- Loud stertor (snoring)
- Frequent awakenings due to gasping or choking
- Nonrefreshing sleep
- Morning headaches

Risk Factors

Obesity, ↑ neck circumference, airway narrowing.

Prevalence

- Most common in middle-aged men and women
- Men: 4%; women: 2%

Treatment

- Positive airway pressure: continuous (CPAP) and in some cases bilevel (BiPAP)
- Behavioral strategies such as weight loss and exercise
- Surgery

Mr. Richards is a 22-year-old college student with a history of dysthymic disorder who arrives at the outpatient psychiatry clinic complaining of daytime sleepiness. He reports that during the past 2 years, he has fallen asleep while in social situations and during his college classes. He often takes naps during class, in movie theaters, and sometimes in the middle of conversations with his girlfriend. His naps typically last for 5–10 minutes and he awakens feeling better. However, within the next 2–3 hours he feels sleepy again. His colleagues joke about his tendency to sleep everywhere, and he feels embarrassed by this.

Mr. Richards also complains of "weird" experiences while sleeping. He reports that he sometimes sees bright colors and hears loud sounds that feel real to him. He says that when this occurs it is difficult to distinguish if he is dreaming or is awake. He feels frightened by these experiences because he is unable to move when they happen. However, after a few minutes he reports that these feelings resolve, and he is able to move and is fully awake.

In performing a thorough history, you learn that he has had episodes during which he has experienced weakness and has dropped objects from his hands while laughing or becoming angry. Last week, his legs buckled and he fell to the ground after his friends surprised him with a surprise birthday party. He denies ever losing consciousness during these episodes, and there have been no reports of witnessed convulsions.

What is this patient's diagnosis?

This patient's symptoms are consistent with a diagnosis of narcolepsy. The classic narcolepsy tetrad consists of excessive daytime sleepiness or "sleep attacks" plus REM-related sleep phenomena including inability to move during the transition from sleep to wakefulness, hypnagogic or hypnopompic hallucinations, or a sudden loss of muscle tone evoked by strong emotion without loss of consciousness (cataplexy). Cataplexy may be mild, affecting only the voice, face, or arms, or generalized, causing patients to fall to the ground, and occurs in 60–100% of those diagnosed with narcolepsy.

What are Mr. Richards's treatment options?

In the treatment of narcolepsy, it is important for patients to schedule daytime naps and to maintain a regular sleep schedule at night. They should get at least 8 hours of sleep and keep consistent times for sleeping and awakening. Pharmacological treatments may include the use of stimulants (methylphenidate) and antidepressants. The stimulant modafinil and sodium oxybate (unrelated to stimulants) are also effective in the treatment of narcolepsy. Sodium oxybate (Xyrem) is particularly effective in the treatment of cataplexy.

Narcolepsy

Narcolepsy is a characterized by excessive daytime sleepiness and falling asleep at inappropriate times.

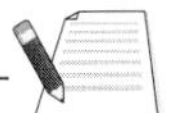

Hypnagogic hallucination: when transitioning *to* sleep

FEATURES

- Irresistible attacks of refreshing sleep that occur daily for at least 3 months
- Cataplexy (brief episodes of sudden bilateral loss of muscle tone, most often associated with intense emotion)
- Hallucinations and/or sleep paralysis at the beginning or end of sleep episodes

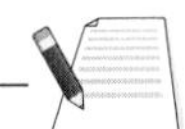

Hypnopompic hallucination: when transitioning *from* sleep

EPIDEMIOLOGY/PREVALENCE

- Narcolepsy with cataplexy occurs in 0.02–0.16% of the U.S. population.
- Males and females are equally affected.

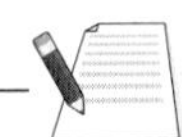

Don't confuse narcoleptic cataplexy with catalepsy (unprovoked muscular rigidity).

PATHOPHYSIOLOGY

- Linked to a loss of hypothalamic neurons that contain hypocretin
- May have autoimmune component

TABLE 14-1. **Circadian Rhythm Sleep Disorders**

Disorder	Definition	Risk Factors	Treatments
Delayed sleep phase disorder (DPSD)	Chronic or recurrent delay in sleep onset and awakening times with preserved quality and duration of sleep	■ Puberty (secondary to temporal changes in melatonin secretion) ■ Caffeine and nicotine use ■ Irregular sleep schedules	■ Timed bright light phototherapy during early morning ■ Administration of melatonin in the evening ■ Chronotherapy (delaying bedtime by a few hours each night)
Advanced sleep phase disorder	Normal duration and quality of sleep with sleep onset and awakening times earlier than desired	Older age	■ Timed bright light phototherapy prior to bedtime ■ Early morning melatonin not recommended (may cause daytime sedation)
Shift-work disorder (SWD)	Sleep deprivation and misalignment of the circadian rhythm secondary to nontraditional work hours	■ Night shift work ■ Rotating shifts ■ Shifts >16 hours ■ *Being a medical/ psychiatry resident*	■ Avoid risk factors ■ Bright light phototherapy to facilitate rapid adaptation to night shift ■ Modafinil may be helpful for patients with severe SWD
Jet lag disorder	Sleep disturbances (insomnia, hypersomnia) associated with travel across multiple time zones	Recent sleep deprivation	Disorder is usually self-limiting. Sleep disturbances generally resolve 2–3 days after travel.

Treatment

- Sleep hygiene
- Scheduled daytime naps
- Avoidance of shift work
- For excessive daytime sleepiness:
  - Amphetamines (D-amphetamine, methamphetamine)
  - Non-amphetamines such as methylphenidate, modafinil, and sodium oxybate
- For cataplexy:
  - Sodium oxybate (drug of choice)
  - Tricyclic antidepressants (TCAs): Imipramine, protriptyline, and clomipramine
  - Selective serotonin reuptake inhibitor (SSRI)/selective serotonin-norepinephrine reuptake inhibitor (SSNRI): Fluoxetine, fluvoxamine, venlafaxine)

Idiopathic Hypersomnia (IH)

Rare disorder characterized by excessive daytime sleepiness, prolonged nocturnal sleep episodes, and frequent irresistible urges to nap. IH can be mild or as debilitating as narcolepsy.

Kleine-Levin Syndrome

A rare disorder characterized by recurrent hypersomnia with episodes of daytime sleepiness with hyperphagia, hypersexuality, and aggression.

Circadian Rhythm Sleep Disorders

Circadian rhythm sleep disorders are caused by either intrinsic defects in the circadian pacemaker or impaired entrainment (absence of light or other time-signaling stimuli). Subtypes include delayed sleep phase disorder, shift-work disorder, and jet lag disorder (see Table 14-1).

Symptoms

- Excessive daytime sleepiness
- Insomnia
- Sleep inertia
- Headaches
- Difficulty concentrating
- ↑ reaction times and frequent performance errors
- Irritability
- Waking up at inappropriate times

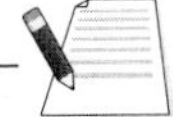

The suprachiasmic nucleus (SCN) in the hypothalamus coordinates 24-hour or circadian rhythmicity.

PARASOMNIAS

- Abnormal behaviors or experiences that occur during sleep and are often associated with sleep disruption.
- Symptoms may include abnormal movements, emotions, dreams, and autonomic activity.
- Common in childhood and adolescence.

Sleepwalking

Features

- Characterized by simple to complex behaviors that are initiated during slow-wave sleep and result in walking during sleep.
- Behaviors may include sitting up in bed, eating, and in some cases "escaping" outdoors.
- Eyes are usually open with a "glassy look."
- Difficulty arousing the sleepwalker during an episode.
- Confusion on awakening, amnesia for episode.
- Episodes usually end with patients returning to bed or awakening confused and disoriented.
- Rare cases associated with violent behavior, especially upon forced awakening.

Epidemiology

- Occurs in 1–4% of adults
- 10–20% in children and adolescents
- Occurs more often in children with obstructive sleep apnea

Risk Factors

- Sleep deprivation
- Irregular sleep schedules
- Stress
- Hyperthyroidism
- Obstructive sleep apnea
- Seizures
- Migraines
- Medications, including sedatives/hypnotics, lithium, and anticholinergics
- Magnesium deficiency

Etiology

- Unknown
- Familial basis in roughly one-third of cases
- Usually not associated with any significant underlying psychiatric or psychological problems

Treatment

- Patients may benefit from addressing precipitating factors, ensuring a safe environment, and proper sleep hygiene.
- Refractory cases may respond to clonazepam, other benzodiazepine receptor agonists, or TCA.

Sleep Terrors

Features

- Episodes of sudden arousal with screaming from slow-wave sleep in what appears to be a state of complete terror.
- Sympathetic hyperactivation, including tachycardia, tachypnea, diaphoresis, and ↑ muscle tone.
- After episode, patients usually return to sleep without awakening.
- Usually amnesic about episode.
- Confused and disoriented upon forced awakening.
- In rare cases, awakening elicits aggressive behavior.

Epidemiology

- Occurs in 1–6% of children and 1–2% of adults.
- Prevalence is greater in first-degree relatives of affected patients.
- High comorbidity with sleepwalking.

Risk Factors

- Fever
- Nocturnal asthma
- Gastroesopohageal reflux disease (GERD)
- Sleep deprivation
- Central nervous system–stimulating medications
- Other sleep disorder such as sleep apnea

TREATMENT

- Reassurance that the condition is benign and self-limited.
- Consider low-dose, short-acting benzodiazepines (clonazepam, diazepam) in adults with refractory cases.
- Sleep hygiene, psychotherapy.

Nightmare Disorder

FEATURES

- Recurrent frightening dreams that tend to terminate in awakening with vivid recall
- No confusion or disorientation upon awakening
- Can → significant distress and anxiety

EPIDEMIOLOGY

- Occurs in 5% of adults, estimated to be higher in women.
- Nightmares are seen in at least 50% of posttraumatic stress disorder (PTSD) cases.

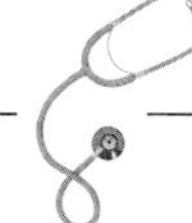

Imagery rehearsal therapy (IRT) has been very successful in treating recurrent nightmares in patients with PTSD.

TREATMENT

- **Imagery rehearsal therapy** (IRT) involves the use of mental imagery to modify the outcome of a recurrent nightmare, writing down the improved outcome, then mentally rehearsing it in a relaxed state.
- Severe cases may benefit from use of antidepressants.

REM Sleep Behavior Disorder (RBD)

FEATURES

- Characterized by muscle atonia during REM sleep and complex motor activity associated with dream mentation (dream enactment).
- Dream-enacting behaviors, which may include:
  - Sleep talking
  - Yelling
  - Limb jerking
  - Walking and/or running
  - Punching and/or other violent behaviors
- Presenting complaint is often violent behaviors during sleep resulting in injury to the patient and/or to the bed partner.

EPIDEMIOLOGY

- Prevalence in general population: 0.5%
- Occurs primarily in males

RISK FACTORS

- Older age, generally between the ages of 60 and 70
- Psychiatric medications such as TCAs, SSRIs, and monoamine oxidase inhibitors (MAOIs)
- Narcolepsy
- Brain stem lesions
- Dementias such as olivopontocerebellar atrophy and diffuse Lewy body disease

Sexual disorders include disturbances of any part of the normal sexual response cycle or pain during intercourse.

SEXUAL RESPONSE CYCLE

There are several stages of normal sexual response in men and women:

1. **Desire:** The interest in sexual activity, often reflected by sexual fantasies.
2. **Excitement:** Begins with either fantasy or physical contact. It is characterized in men by erections and in women by vaginal lubrication, clitoral erection, labial swelling, and elevation of the uterus in the pelvis *(tenting)*. Both men and women experience nipple erection and increased pulse and blood pressure.
3. **Plateau:** Characterized in men by ↑ size of the testicles, tightening of the scrotal sac, and secretion of a few drops of seminal fluid. Women experience contraction of the outer one-third of the vagina and enlargement of the upper one-third of the vagina. Facial flushing and ↑ in pulse, blood pressure, and respiration occur in both men and women.
4. **Orgasm:** Men ejaculate and women have contractions of the uterus and lower one-third of the vagina.
5. **Resolution:** Muscles relax and cardiovascular state returns to baseline. Men have a *refractory period* during which they cannot re-experience orgasm; women have little or no refractory period.

SEXUAL CHANGES WITH AGING

The desire for sexual activity does not usually change as people age. However, men usually require more direct stimulation of genitals and more time to achieve orgasm. The intensity of ejaculation usually ↓, and the length of refractory period ↑.

After menopause, women experience vaginal dryness and thinning due to ↓ levels of estrogen. These conditions can be treated with hormone replacement therapy or vaginal creams.

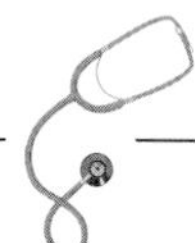

Alcohol and marijuana enhance sexual desire by suppressing inhibitions. However, long-term alcohol use **decreases** sexual desire. Cocaine and amphetamines enhance libido by stimulating dopamine receptors. Narcotics inhibit libido.

DIFFERENTIAL DIAGNOSIS OF SEXUAL DYSFUNCTION

Problems with sexual functioning may be due to any of the following:

- General medical conditions: Examples include history of atherosclerosis (causing erectile dysfunction from vascular occlusion), diabetes (causing erectile dysfunction from vascular changes and peripheral neuropathy), and pelvic adhesions (causing dyspareunia in women).
- Medication side effects: Antihypertensives, anticholinergics, antidepressants (especially selective serotonin reuptake inhibitors [SSRIs]), and antipsychotics may contribute to sexual dysfunction.
- Depression.
- Substance abuse.

- Abnormal levels of gonadal hormones:
  - **Estrogen:** ↓ levels after menopause cause vaginal dryness and thinning in women (without affecting desire).
  - **Testosterone:** Promotes libido (desire) in both men and women.
  - **Progesterone:** Inhibits libido in both men and women by blocking androgen receptors; found in oral contraceptives, hormone replacement therapy, and treatments for prostate cancer.
- Presence of a sexual disorder (see below).

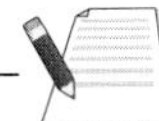

Dopamine enhances libido. Serotonin inhibits sexual function.

SEXUAL DISORDERS

Sexual disorders are problems involving any stage of the sexual response cycle. They all share the following *Diagnostic and Statistical Manual of Mental Disorders*, 4th ed., Text Revision (DSM-IV-TR) criteria:

- The disorder causes marked distress or interpersonal difficulty.
- The dysfunction is not caused by substance use or a general medical condition.

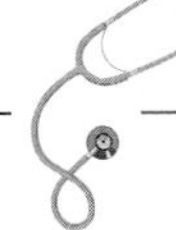

Causes of sexual disorders may be physiological or psychological. Psychological causes of sexual disorders are usually comorbid with other psychiatric disorders, such as depression or anxiety.

Mr. Jones is a 58-year-old married man with a history of major depressive disorder who arrives at your outpatient clinic for a 6-month follow up visit. He complains of recent marital problems with his wife of 30 years. He is being treated with an SSRI, and his depressive symptoms have been stable for over 2 years on his current dose. Upon further questioning, he reveals that he has been having sex with his wife less often than usual, "only once or twice a month." He states that this is a marked decrease since his last visit with you. He feels that lately they have been arguing more and feels that their decrease in sexual activity has adversely affected their [illegible] energy.

Mr. Jones denies having urges to masturbate in the times between sexual intercourse with his wife. He also denies having any affairs, laughing nervously while saying, "I can barely satisfy my own wife." He appears sad and states that he is beginning to feel "down" about this. When he does have sex, he reports that it is initiated by his wife, and he is initially reluctant to engage in sexual activity. However, once he does, he denies any problems with having or sustaining an erection and denies any difficulties in reaching orgasm. Mr. Jones reports that he drinks two or three drinks per day on the weekends, and he does not use any recreational drugs.

What is his most likely diagnosis? What other considerations should be made?

The patient's most likely diagnosis is hypoactive sexual desire disorder. Although more prevalent in women, this diagnosis should not be overlooked in men. As this clinical case shows, the patient does not seem to fantasize or desire sexual activity despite prior history of doing so. He appears distressed by this and reports that it is causing interpersonal dysfunction. Although his depression has remained stable during the past 2 years and the patient does not report symptoms that would suggest a current depressive episode, his sexual complaints and fatigue symptoms might suggest a relapse of depressive symptoms and should be

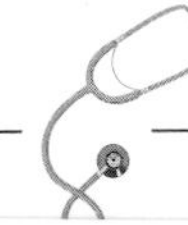

Problems with sexual desire may be due to stress, hostility toward a partner, poor self-esteem, abstinence from sex for a prolonged period, or unconscious fears about sex.

(continued)

monitored closely. It is also important to consider if his treatment with an SSRI is affecting his sexual functioning.

What should you consider in the initial management of this patient's complaints?

His initial management should consist of a thorough history, a physical examination, and laboratory tests (testosterone levels, thyroid stimulating hormone levels) that might rule out endocrine abnormalities. Treatment considerations should include outpatient psychotherapy, dual-sex therapy, behavior therapy, or group therapy.

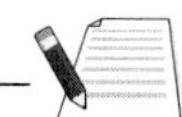

The most common sexual disorders in women are sexual desire disorder and orgasmic disorder. The most common disorders in men are secondary erectile disorder and premature ejaculation.

Disorders of Desire

- **Hypoactive sexual desire disorder:** Absence or deficiency of sexual desire or fantasies (occurs in up to 20% of general population and is more common in women)
- **Sexual aversion disorder:** Avoidance of genital contact with a sexual partner

Disorders of Arousal (Excitement)

Stress, fear, fatigue, anxiety, and feelings of guilt may contribute to both erectile disorder in men and sexual arousal disorder in women.

- **Male erectile disorder:** Inability to attain an erection. Commonly referred to as *impotence*. May be *primary* (never had one) or *secondary* (acquired after previous ability to maintain erections). Men who have erections in the morning, during masturbation, or with other sexual partners usually have a psychological rather than physical etiology.
- **Female sexual arousal disorder:** Inability to maintain lubrication until completion of sex act (high prevalence—up to 33% of women)

Disorders of Orgasm

Both male and female orgasmic disorders may be either *primary* (never achieved orgasm) or *secondary* (acquired). Causes may include relationship problems, guilt, stress, and so on.

- **Female orgasmic disorder:** Inability to have an orgasm after a normal excitement phase. The estimated prevalence in women is 30%.
- **Male orgasmic disorder:** Achieves orgasm with great difficulty, if at all; much lower incidence than impotence or premature ejaculation. Estimated prevalence in men is 5%.
- **Premature ejaculation:** Ejaculation earlier than desired time (before or immediately upon entering the vagina). High prevalence—up to 35% of all male sexual disorders.

Sexual Pain Disorders

- **Dyspareunia:** Genital pain before, during, or after sexual intercourse; much higher incidence in women than men; often associated with vaginismus (see below)
- **Vaginismus:** Involuntary muscle contraction of the outer third of the vagina during insertion of penis or object (such as speculum or tampon); ↑ incidence in higher socioeconomic groups and in women of strict religious upbringing

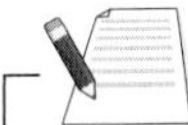

Other DSM-IV-TR categories of sexual dysfunction include substance-induced dysfunction, dysfunction due to general medical condition, or dysfunction not otherwise specified.

TREATMENT OF SEXUAL DISORDERS

Dual Sex Therapy

Dual sex therapy utilizes the concept of the marital unit, rather than the individual, as the target of therapy. Couples meet with a male and female therapist together in four-way sessions to identify and discuss their sexual problems. Therapists suggest sexual exercises for the couple to attempt at home; activities initially focus on heightening sensory awareness and progressively incorporate ↑ levels of sexual contact. Treatment is short term. This therapy is most useful when no other psychopathology is involved.

Behavior Therapy

Behavior therapy approaches sexual dysfunction as a learned maladaptive behavior. It utilizes traditional therapies such as systematic desensitization, where patients are progressively exposed to increasing levels of stimuli that provoke their anxiety. Eventually, patients are able to respond appropriately to the stimuli. Other forms of behavioral therapy may include muscle relaxation techniques, assertiveness training, and prescribed sexual exercises to try at home.

Hypnosis

Most often used adjunctively with other therapies. Most useful if anxiety is present.

Group Therapy

May be used as primary or adjunctive therapy.

Analytically Oriented Psychotherapy

Individual, long-term therapy that focuses on feelings, fears, dreams, and interpersonal problems that may be contributing to sexual disorder.

Pharmacologic Treatment

- **Erectile disorder:** Phosphodiesterase-5 inhibitors (eg, sildenafil is given orally and enhance blood flow to the penis); they require sexual stimulation to achieve an erection. Alprostadil, injected into the corpora cavernosa or transurethral, acts locally; it produces an erection within 2–3 minutes and works in the absence of sexual stimulation.
- **Premature ejaculation:** SSRIs and tricyclic antidepressants (TCAs) prolong the time from stimulation to orgasm.
- **Hypoactive sexual desire disorder:** Testosterone as replacement therapy for men with low levels. Low doses may also improve libido in women. Estrogen replacement may improve vaginal dryness and atrophy in hypoestrogenemic women.

Mechanical Therapies

- **Male erectile disorder:** Vacuum pumps, constrictive rings, or surgical insertion of semirigid or inflatable tubes into the corpora cavernosa (used only for end-stage impotence).
- **Male orgasmic disorder:** Gradual progression from extravaginal ejaculation (via masturbation) to intravaginal.
- **Female orgasmic disorder:** Masturbation (sometimes with vibrator).
- **Premature ejaculation:**
  - The *squeeze technique* is used to ↑ the threshold of excitability. When the man has been excited to near ejaculation, he or his sexual partner is instructed to squeeze the glans of his penis in order to prevent ejaculation. Gradually, he gains awareness about his sexual sensations and learns to achieve greater ejaculatory control.
  - The *stop-start technique* involves cessation of all penile stimulation when the man is near ejaculation. This technique functions in the same manner as the squeeze technique.
- **Dyspareunia:** Gradual desensitization to achieve intercourse, starting with muscle relaxation techniques, progressing to erotic massage, and finally achieving sexual intercourse.
- **Vaginismus:** Women may obtain some relief by dilating their vaginas regularly with their fingers or a dilator.

PARAPHILIAS

Paraphilias are sexual disorders characterized by engagement in unusual sexual activities and/or preoccupation with unusual sexual urges or fantasies for at least 6 months that cause impairment in daily functioning. Paraphilic fantasies alone are not considered disorders unless they are intense, recurrent, and interfere with daily life; occasional fantasies are considered normal components of sexuality (even if unusual).

Only a small percentage of people suffer from paraphilias. Most paraphilias occur only in men, but sadism, masochism, and pedophilia may also occur in women. The most common paraphilias are pedophilia, voyeurism, and exhibitionism.

Examples of Paraphilias

- **Pedophilia:** Sexual gratification from fantasies or behaviors involving sexual acts with children age 13 years or younger. DSM-IV-TR specifies that the person is at least age 16 and at least 5 years older than the child.
- **Frotteurism:** Sexual pleasure from touching or rubbing against a nonconsenting person.
- **Voyeurism:** Watching unsuspecting nude individuals (often with binoculars) in order to obtain sexual pleasure.
- **Exhibitionism:** Exposure of one's genitals to strangers.
- **Sadism:** Sexual excitement from hurting or humiliating another.
- **Fetishism:** Sexual preference for inanimate objects (eg, shoes or pantyhose).
- **Transvestic fetishism:** Sexual gratification in men (usually heterosexual) from wearing women's clothing (especially underwear).
- **Masochism:** Sexual excitement from being humiliated or beaten.
- **Necrophilia:** Sexual pleasure from engaging in sexual activity with dead people.
- **Telephone scatologia:** Sexual excitement from calling unsuspecting women and engaging in sexual conversations with them.

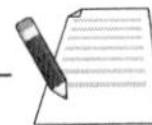

The three most common types of paraphilia: pedophilia, voyeurism, exhibitionism.

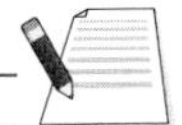

Aversion therapy is a common treatment for paraphilias (as well as some substance abuse).

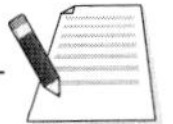

An example of fetishism is a man being sexually aroused by women's shoes.

COURSE AND PROGNOSIS

- *Poor prognostic factors* are early age of onset, comorbid substance abuse, high frequency of behavior, and referral by law enforcement agencies (after arrest).
- *Good prognostic factors* are self-referral for treatment, sense of guilt associated with the behavior, and history of otherwise normal sexual activity in addition to the paraphilia.

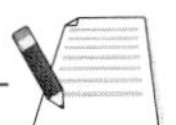

An example of transvestic fetishism is a person being sexually aroused by dressing up as a member of the opposite gender. This does *not* mean they are homosexual.

TREATMENT

- **Insight-oriented psychotherapy:** Most common method. Patients gain insight into the stimuli that cause them to act as they do.
- **Behavior therapy:** Aversive conditioning used to disrupt the learned abnormal behavior by coupling the impulse with an unpleasant stimulus such as an electric shock.
- **Pharmacologic therapy:** Antiandrogens have been used to treat hypersexual paraphilias in men by reducing sexual desire.

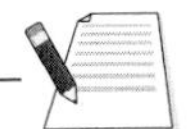

Most rape offenders are usually relatives of the victim.

GENDER IDENTITY DISORDER

Gender identity disorder is commonly referred to as *transsexuality*. People with this disorder have the subjective feeling that they were born the wrong sex. They may dress as the opposite sex, take sex hormones, or undergo sex change operations.

Cross-gender behaviors in children with this disorder often begin before age 3, the time when gender identity is established. Adults in whom the disorder is first diagnosed usually have experienced some feelings of gender discomfort from early childhood, although the history is often vague.

Gender identity disorder is often associated with psychological comorbidities such as major depression, anxiety disorders, and suicide.

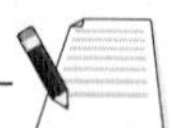

Transsexuals identify themselves more with the opposite sex and commonly undergo surgery to morphologically appear like the opposite sex.

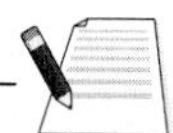

If someone experiences severe distress and depressive symptoms because of the conflict between their homosexuality and the values of society, they may have *adjustment disorder* or *major depressive disorder.* This is not a sexual disorder.

DIAGNOSIS AND DSM-IV-TR CRITERIA

1. A strong and persistent cross-gender identification
2. Persistent discomfort with his or her sex or sense of inappropriateness in the gender role of that sex
3. Clinical distress or impairment in social, occupational, or other important areas of functioning

TREATMENT

Therapy, family involvement for younger patients, and possibly sex reassignment by hormonal and surgical techniques for adults.

HOMOSEXUALITY (NOT A DISORDER!)

Homosexuality is a sexual or romantic desire for people of the same sex. ***It is not a sexual disorder and is a normal variant of sexual orientation.*** Its true incidence is unknown because of the unreliability of interview data, but it occurs < 10% in both sexes. The etiology of homosexuality is unknown.

Prepubertal same-sex exploratory activities are common and do not signify latent homosexuality.

HIGH-YIELD FACTS IN

Psychotherapies

It is common to combine psychotherapy with medications. *Split treatment* describes the arrangement for a psychiatrist to prescribe medication and someone else provides therapy. The psychiatrist and therapist should regularly discuss together the patient's treatment.

PSYCHOANALYSIS AND RELATED THERAPIES

Psychoanalysis is not indicated for people who have problems with reality testing, such as psychotic patients, or people with severe cluster A and B personality disorders.

Psychoanalysis and its related therapies are derived from Sigmund Freud's psychoanalytic theories of the mind. Freud proposed that behaviors, or symptoms, result from *unconscious* mental processes, including defense mechanisms and conflicts between one's ego, id, superego, and external reality. Since the time of Freud, many other psychoanalytic theories have been developed. Influential theorists have included Melanie Klein, Heinz Kohut, Michael Balint, Margaret Mahler, and others.

Examples of psychoanalytic therapies include:

- Psychoanalysis
- Psychoanalytically oriented psychotherapy
- Brief dynamic therapy
- Interpersonal therapy

FREUD'S THEORIES OF THE MIND

Normal development: **Id** is present at birth, **ego** develops after birth, **superego** development begins at age 6.

Topographic Theory

1. **Unconscious:** Includes repressed thoughts that are out of one's awareness; involves *primary process* thinking (primitive, pleasure-seeking urges with no regard to logic or time, prominent in children and psychotics). Thoughts and ideas may be repressed into the unconscious because they are embarrassing, shameful, or otherwise too painful.
2. **Preconscious:** Contains memories that are easy to bring into awareness, but not unless consciously retrieved.
3. **Conscious:** Involves current thoughts and secondary process thinking (logical, organized, mature, and can delay gratification).

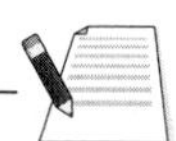

According to Freud, the superego is the aspect of one's psyche that represents "morality, society, and parental teaching."

Structural Theory

1. **Id:** Unconscious; involves instinctual sexual/aggressive urges and primary process thinking.
2. **Ego:** Serves as a mediator between the id and external environment and seeks to develop satisfying interpersonal relationships; uses *defense mechanisms* (see below) to control instinctual urges and distinguishes fantasy from reality using *reality testing.* Problems with reality testing occur in psychotic individuals.
3. **Superego:** Moral conscience.

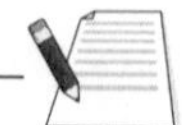

Operating a washing machine can be considered an example of "executive functioning."

Defense mechanisms are used by the ego to protect oneself and relieve anxiety by keeping conflicts out of awareness. They are *unconscious* processes that may be normal and healthy when used in moderation (ie, adaptive), or they may be unhealthy and seen in some psychiatric disorders when used excessively (ie, maladaptive).

Defense mechanisms are often classified hierarchically. **Mature** defense mechanisms are healthy and adaptive, and they are seen in normal adults. **Neurotic** defenses are encountered in obsessive-compulsive patients, hysterical patients, and adults under stress. **Immature** defenses are seen in children, adolescents, psychotic patients, and some nonpsychotic patients. They are the most primitive defense mechanisms.

Mature Defenses

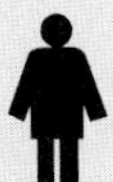

A former street thug becomes a social worker to help reform kids in gangs. *What is the defense mechanism?* Sublimation—the channeling of destructive impulses to create something constructive.

Mature ego defenses are commonly found in healthy, high-functioning adults. These defenses often help people integrate conflicting emotions and thoughts.

1. **Altruism:** Performing acts that benefit others in order to vicariously experience pleasure. (*Clinical example:* A patient's child recently died from ovarian cancer. As part of the grieving process, the patient donates money to help raise community awareness about the symptoms of ovarian cancer so other patients could potentially benefit from early intervention.)
2. **Humor:** Expressing (usually) unpleasant or uncomfortable feelings without causing discomfort to self or others.
3. **Sublimation:** Satisfying socially objectionable impulses in an acceptable manner (thus *channeling* them rather than *preventing* them). (*Clinical example:* Person with unconscious urges to physically control others becomes a prison guard.)
4. **Suppression:** Purposely ignoring an unacceptable impulse or emotion in order to diminish discomfort and accomplish a task. (*Clinical example:* Nurse who feels nauseated by an infected wound puts aside feelings of disgust to clean wound and provide necessary patient care.)

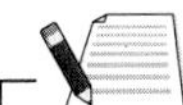

Thought suppression, as a defense mechanism, is a *conscious* process that involves avoiding paying attention to a particular emotion. Therefore, it is *not* an unconscious reaction.

Neurotic Defenses

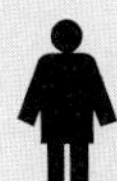

A man buys himself an expensive new watch and tells his friends that he needed it because his old one was not reliable enough and he needs to make sure to get to his appointments on time. *Think: Rationalization.*

1. **Controlling:** Regulating situations and events of external environment to relieve anxiety.

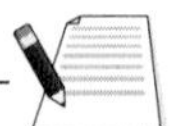

Intellectualization is a defense mechanism where reasoning is used to block confrontation with an unconscious conflict. It is associated emotional stress.

2. **Displacement:** Shifting emotions from an undesirable situation to one that is personally tolerable. (*Clinical example:* Student who is angry at his mother talks back to his teacher the next day and refuses to obey her instructions.)
3. **Intellectualization:** Avoiding negative feelings by excessive use of intellectual functions and by focusing on irrelevant details or inanimate objects. (*Clinical example:* Physician dying from colon cancer describes the pathophysiology of his disease in detail to his 12-year-old son.)
4. **Isolation of affect:** Unconsciously limiting the experience of feelings or emotions associated with a stressful life event in order to avoid anxiety. (*Clinical example:* Woman describes the recent death of her beloved husband without emotion.)
5. **Rationalization:** Creating explanations of an event in order to justify outcomes or behaviors and to make them acceptable. (*Clinical example:* "My boss fired me today because she's short tempered and impulsive, not because I haven't done a good job.")
6. **Reaction formation:** Doing the opposite of an unacceptable impulse. (*Clinical example:* Man who is in love with his married coworker insults her.)
7. **Repression:** Preventing a thought or feeling from entering consciousness. (Repression is unconscious, whereas suppression is a conscious act.)

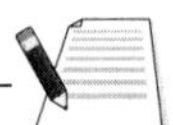

A man who regularly steals money from his roommate, who constantly suspects his roommate is stealing from him, is an example of **projection.**

Immature Defenses

1. **Acting out:** Giving in to an impulse, even if socially inappropriate, in order to avoid the anxiety of suppressing that impulse. (*Clinical example:* Man who has been told his therapist is going on vacation "forgets" his last appointment and skips it.)
2. **Denial:** Not accepting reality that is too painful (*Clinical example:* Woman who has been scheduled for a breast mass biopsy cancels her appointment because she believes she is healthy.)
3. **Regression:** Performing behaviors from an earlier stage of development in order to avoid tension associated with current phase of development. (*Clinical example:* Woman brings her childhood teddy bear to the hospital when she has to spend the night.)
4. **Projection:** Attributing objectionable thoughts or emotions to others. (*Clinical example:* Husband who is attracted to other women believes his wife is having an affair.)

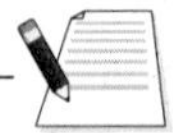

The Freudian superego represents society and societal norms.

Other Defense Mechanisms

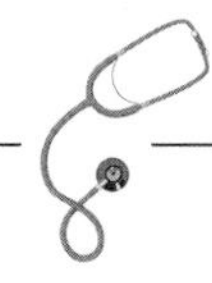

Beware when your patient thinks you're so cool to talk to but hates the "evil attending." That's **splitting.**

1. **Splitting:** Labeling people as all good or all bad (often seen in borderline personality disorder). (*Clinical example:* Woman who tells her doctor, "You and the nurses are the only people who understand me; all the other doctors are mean and impatient.")
2. **Undoing:** Attempting to reverse a situation by adopting a new behavior. (*Clinical example:* Man who has had a brief fantasy of killing his wife by sabotaging her car takes the car in for a complete checkup.)

PSYCHOANALYSIS

The goal of psychoanalysis is to resolve *unconscious conflicts* by bringing repressed experiences and feelings into awareness and integrating them into the patient's conscious experience. Psychoanalysis is therefore *insight oriented.* Patients best suited for psychoanalysis have the following characteristics: under age 40, not psychotic, intelligent, and stable in relationships and daily living. Treatment is usually 4–5 days per week for multiple years. During therapy sessions, the patient usually lies on a couch with the therapist seated out of view.

To become an analyst, doctors (MDs, PhDs, and sometimes PsyDs and MSWs) must complete training at a psychoanalytic institute. In addition to attending seminars and treating patients under supervision, the training typically requires that trainees receive their own analysis.

Psychoanalysis may be useful in the treatment of:

- Cluster C personality disorders
- Anxiety disorders
- Obsessive-compulsive disorder
- Problems coping with life events
- Anorexia nervosa
- Sexual disorders
- Dysthymic disorder

Important Concepts and Techniques Used in Psychoanalysis

- **Free association:** The patient is asked to say whatever comes into his or her mind during therapy sessions. The purpose is to bring forth thoughts and feelings from the unconscious so that the therapist may interpret them.
- **Dream interpretation:** Dreams are seen to represent conflict between urges and fears. Interpretation of dreams by the psychoanalyst is used to help achieve therapeutic goals.
- **Therapeutic alliance:** This is the bond between the therapist and the patient, who work together toward a therapeutic goal.
- **Transference:** Projection of unconscious feelings about important figures in the patient's life onto the therapist. Interpretation of transference is used to help the patient gain insight and resolve unconscious conflict.
- **Countertransference:** Projection of unconscious feelings about important figures in the therapist's life onto the patient. The therapist must remain aware of countertransference issues, as they may interfere with his or her objectivity.

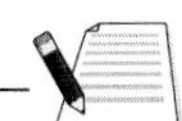

An example of transference would be when a patient who has repressed feelings of abandonment by her father becomes angry when her therapist is late for the appointment.

Psychoanalysis-Related Therapies

Examples of psychoanalysis-related therapies include:

1. **Psychoanalytically oriented psychotherapy** and **brief dynamic psychotherapy:** These employ similar techniques and theories as psychoanalysis, but they are briefer (weekly sessions for 6 months to $1\frac{1}{2}$ years) and involve face-to-face sessions between the therapist and patient (no couch).

2. **Interpersonal therapy:** Focuses on development of social skills to help treat certain psychiatric disorders. Treatment is short (once-weekly sessions for 3–6 months). The idea is to improve interpersonal relations. Sessions may also focus on reassurance, clarification of emotions, improving interpersonal communication, and testing perceptions.
3. **Supportive psychotherapy:** Purpose is to help patient feel safe during a difficult time. Ideal patients are healthy individuals who are in crisis. Treatment is not insight oriented but instead focuses on empathy, understanding, and education. Supportive therapy is commonly used as adjunctive treatment in even the most severe mental disorders. Helps to build up the patient's healthy defenses.

BEHAVIORAL THERAPY

Behavioral therapy, largely pioneered by B. F. Skinner, seeks to treat psychiatric disorders by helping patients change behaviors that contribute to their symptoms. It can be used to extinguish maladaptive behaviors (such as phobic avoidance, sexual dysfunction, compulsions, etc) by replacing them with healthy alternatives. Time course depends on the situation.

Learning Theory

Behavioral therapy is based on **learning theory,** which states that behaviors can be learned by *conditioning* and can similarly be unlearned by *deconditioning.*

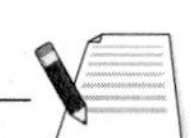

Positive reinforcement: Giving a reward for a desired behavior.

Conditioning

- **Classical conditioning:** A stimulus can eventually evoke a conditioned response. (*Example:* Pavlov's dog would salivate when hearing a bell because the dog had learned that bells were always followed by food.)
- **Operant conditioning:** Behaviors can be learned when followed by positive or negative *reinforcement.* (*Example:* Skinner's box—a rat happened upon a lever and received food; eventually, it learned to press the lever for food [trial-and-error learning].)

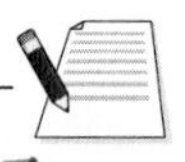

Negative reinforcement: Encouraging a behavior by removing an aversive stimulus. Punishment is an aversive response to a behavior. Punishment is *not* negative reinforcement.

Behavioral Therapy Techniques (Deconditioning)

- **Systemic desensitization:** The patient performs relaxation techniques while being exposed to increasing doses of an anxiety-provoking stimulus. Gradually, he or she learns to associate the stimulus with a state of relaxation. Commonly used to treat phobic disorders. (*Example:* A patient who has a fear of spiders is first shown a photograph of a spider, followed by exposure to a stuffed toy spider, then a videotape of a spider, and finally a live spider. At each step, the patient learns to relax while exposed to an increasing dose of the phobia.)
- **Flooding and implosion:** Through habituation, the patient is confronted with a real (flooding) or imagined (implosion) anxiety-provoking stimulus and not allowed to withdraw from it until he or she feels calm and in control. Relaxation exercises are used to help the patient

tolerate the stimulus. Commonly used to treat phobic disorders. (*Example:* A patient who has a fear of flying is made to fly in an airplane [flooding] or imagine flying [implosion].)

- **Aversion therapy:** A negative stimulus (such as an electric shock) is repeatedly paired with a specific behavior to create an unpleasant response. Commonly used to treat addictions or paraphilias. (*Example:* An alcoholic patient is prescribed Antabuse, which makes him ill every time he drinks alcohol.)
- **Token economy:** Rewards are given after specific behaviors to positively reinforce them. Commonly used to encourage showering, shaving, and other positive behaviors in disorganized or mentally retarded individuals.
- **Biofeedback:** Physiological data (such as heart rate and blood pressure measurements) are given to patients as they try to mentally control physiological states. Commonly used to treat migraines, hypertension, chronic pain, asthma, and incontinence. (*Example:* A patient is given her heart rate and blood pressure measurements during a migraine while being instructed to mentally control visceral changes that affect her pain.)

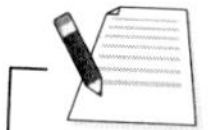

Biofeedback used to treat a wide scope of clinical conditions including agoraphobia, fecal incontinence, tension headache, and hypertension.

COGNITIVE THERAPY

Cognitive therapy, pioneered by Aaron T. Beck, seeks to correct faulty assumptions and negative feelings that exacerbate psychiatric symptoms. The patient is taught to identify maladaptive thoughts and replace them with positive ones. Most commonly used to treat depressive and anxiety disorders. May also be used for paranoid personality disorder, obsessive-compulsive disorder, somatoform disorders, and eating disorders. Cognitive therapy can be more effective than medication.

Clinical Example of the Cognitive Theory of Depression

- **Faulty assumptions,** also known as **cognitive distortions** (*Example:* If I were smart, I would do well on tests. I must not be smart since I received average grades this semester.)
- → **Negative thoughts** (*Example:* I am stupid. I will never amount to anything worthwhile. Nobody likes a worthless person.)
- → **Psychopathology:** Depression.

COGNITIVE-BEHAVIORAL THERAPY (CBT)

CBT combines ideas from cognitive therapy and behavior therapy. Treatment follows a protocol or manual with homework assignments between therapy sessions. During therapy sessions, the patient and therapist set an **agenda,** review homework, and challenge cognitive distortions. The patient learns how his behavior is influenced by his thoughts. Treatment is usually brief and may last from 6 weeks to 6 months. Research has shown that CBT is effective for many psychiatric illnesses, including depression, anxiety, and substance abuse.

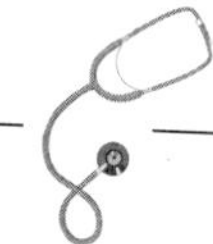

CBT focuses on a patient's current symptoms and problems by examining the connection between thoughts and behaviors.

HIGH-YIELD FACTS
PSYCHOTHERAPIES

Other Treatments

SIDE EFFECTS IN A NUTSHELL

1. **HAM side effects** (*antiHistamine*—sedation, weight gain; *antiAdrenergic*—hypotension; *antiMuscarinic*—dry mouth, blurred vision, urinary retention). Found in tricyclic antidepressants (TCAs) and low-potency antipsychotics.
2. **Serotonin syndrome:** Confusion, flushing, diaphoresis, tremor, myoclonic jerks, hyperthermia, hypertonicity, rhabdomyolysis, renal failure, and death.
   - Occurs when there is too much serotonin, classically when selective serotonin reuptake inhibitors (SSRIs) and monoamine oxidase inhibitors (MAOIs) are combined
   - Treatment: Stop drugs
3. **Hypertensive crisis:** Caused by a buildup of stored catecholamines. MAOIs plus foods with tyramine (red wine, cheese, chicken liver, cured meats) or plus sympathomimetics.
4. **Extrapyramidal side effects (EPS):** *Parkinsonism*—masklike face, cogwheel rigidity, pill-rolling tremor; *akathisia*—restlessness and agitation; *dystonia*—sustained contraction of muscles of neck, tongue, eyes, diaphragm.
   - Occurs with high-potency traditional antipsychotics
   - Reversible
   - Occurs within *days* of starting med
   - Can be life threatening (eg, dystonia of the diaphragm causing asphyxiation)
5. **Hyperprolactinemia:** Occurs with high-potency traditional antipsychotics and risperidone.
6. **Tardive dyskinesia:** Choreoathetoid muscle movements, usually of mouth and tongue.
   - Occurs after *years* of antipsychotic use (particularly high-potency typical antipsychotics)
   - Can be irreversible
7. **Neuroleptic malignant syndrome:** Fever, tachycardia, hypertension, tremor, elevated creatine phosphokinase (CPK), "lead pipe" rigidity.
   - Can be caused by all antipsychotics after short or long time (↑ with high-potency traditional antipsychotics)
   - A medical emergency with 20% mortality rate
8. **Drug interactions:** *Cytochrome P450* is a group of enzymes in the liver that metabolize many common drugs, including psychiatric drugs.
   - Some drugs *induce* the system, which means that they make the system metabolize drugs faster—drug levels *decrease*.
   - Some drugs *inhibit* the system, which mean that they make the system metabolize drugs more slowly—drug levels *increase*.
   - Common cytochrome P450 enzymes important in metabolizing psychiatric drugs include CYP3A4, CYP2D6, CYP1A2, CYP2C9, CYP2C19.
   - Important CYP450 *inducers* include:
     - Smoking (1A2)
     - Carbamazepine (1A2, 2C9, 3A4)
     - Barbiturates (2C9)
     - St. John's wort (2C19, 3A4)

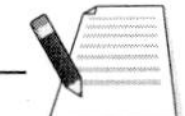

The choice of drug to treat the extrapyramidal symptoms produced by neuroleptics is benzotropine.

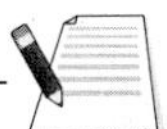

Keeping the "kinesias" (impairment of body function) straight:

- **Tardive dyskinesia** is characterized by grimacing and tongue protrusion.
- **Acute dystonia** is usually characterized by twisting and abnormal postures.
- **Akathisia** is characterized by the inability to sit still.
- **Bradykinesia** is characterized by ↓ or slow body movement.

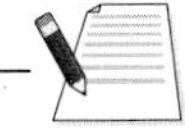

Constipation is common a side effect of anticholinergics.

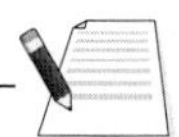

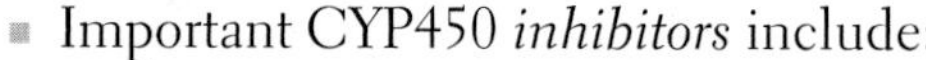

Anticholinergics are known to exacerbate Alzheimer disease.

- Important CYP450 *inhibitors* include:
  - Fluvoxamine (1A2, 2D6, 3A4)
  - Fluoxetine (2C19, 2C9, 2D6)
  - Paroxetine (2D6)
  - Duloxetine (2D6)
  - Sertraline (2C19)

ANTIDEPRESSANTS

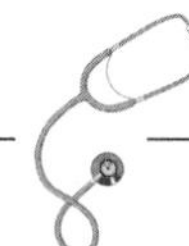

You should give a patient an adequate trial of antidepressant, usually between 1 and 2 months at full dose, before considering changing medications.

- The major categories of antidepressants are:
  - Selective serotonin reuptake inhibitors (SSRIs)
  - Heterocyclic antidepressants, including TCAs and tetracyclic antidepressants
  - Monoamine oxidase inhibitors (MAOIs)
  - Miscellaneous antidepressants
- All antidepressants have similar response rates in treating major depression but differ in safety and side effect profiles.
- About 70% of patients with major depression will respond to antidepressant medication. About 30% of this is placebo response.
- Most antidepressants require a trial of at least 3–4 weeks for effect, with some people requiring as little as 1–2 weeks and some 6–8 weeks for noticeable effects.
- Most antidepressants have a *withdrawal phenomenon*, characterized by dizziness, headaches, nausea, insomnia, and malaise. Depending on the dose and half-life, they may need to be tapered.
- Because of their safety and tolerability, SSRIs and related antidepressants have become the most common agents used to treat major depression. However, the choice of a particular medication used for a given patient should be made based on:
  - Patient's symptoms
  - Previous treatment responses by the patient or a family member to a particular drug
  - Medication side effect profile
  - Comorbid conditions
  - Risk of suicide
  - Cost

Selective Serotonin Reuptake Inhibitors (SSRIs)

- SSRIs inhibit presynaptic serotonin pumps that take up serotonin, → ↑ availability of serotonin in synaptic clefts. However, research indicates that the mechanism of action may be more complex.
- Although their structural differences are minimal, patients often respond differently, in terms of both efficacy and side effects, to different SSRIs.
- Based on their half-lives, most SSRIs can be dosed daily. Fluoxetine also has a weekly dosing form available.
- There is no correlation between plasma levels and efficacy or side effects.

- They are the most commonly prescribed antidepressants due to several distinct advantages:
  - Low incidence of side effects, most of which resolve with time
  - No food restrictions
  - Much safer in overdose
- Examples of SSRIs include:
  - **Fluoxetine (Prozac):**
    - Longest half-life with active metabolites; therefore, no need to taper
    - Safe in pregnancy, approved for use in children
    - More common sleep changes and anxiety
    - Can elevate levels of neuroleptics, leading to ↑ side effects
  - **Sertraline (Zoloft):**
    - Highest risk for gastrointestinal (GI) disturbances
    - Very few drug interactions
    - More common sleep changes
  - **Paroxetine (Paxil):**
    - Highly protein bound, → several drug interactions
    - More anticholinergic effects like sedation, constipation, weight gain
    - Short half-life leading to *withdrawal phenomena* if not taken consistently
  - **Fluvoxamine (Luvox):**
    - Currently approved only for use in obsessive-compulsive disorder (OCD)
    - Nausea and vomiting more common
    - Lots of drug interactions
  - **Citalopram (Celexa):**
    - Fewest drug-drug interactions
    - Possibly fewer sexual side effects
  - **Escitalopram (Lexapro):**
    - Levo-enantiomer of citalopram; similar efficacy, possibly fewer side effects
    - More expensive than citalopram

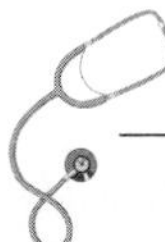

Drugs that ↑ serotonin may be found in over-the-counter cold remedies, possibly → **serotonin syndrome.** A classic example is someone on a high-dose antidepressant taking cough medicine.

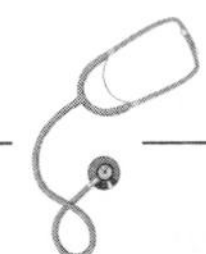

The sexual side effects of SSRIs can be treated by augmenting the regimen with buproprion, changing to a non-SSRI antidepressant, or by adding medications like sildenafil for men.

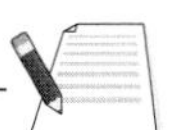

The FDA has a **Black Box Warning** against all SSRIs for "increased suicidal thinking and behavior." This is most documented in children and adolescents, but may be accurate for adults as well.

OCD:
1) SSRI
2) Clomipramine

SIDE EFFECTS

- SSRIs have significantly fewer side effects than TCAs and MAOIs due to serotonin selectivity (they do not act on histamine, adrenergic, or muscarinic receptors).
- In addition, they are much safer in overdose. Most side effects occur because of the extensive number of serotonin receptors throughout the body, including the GI tract.
- Side effects of SSRIs mostly resolve within a few weeks and include:
  - Sexual dysfunction (25–30%): ↓ interest, anorgasmia, delayed ejaculation. These typically do not resolve in a few weeks.
  - GI disturbance: Mostly nausea and diarrhea; giving with food can help.
  - Insomnia: Also vivid dreams, often resolves over time.
  - Headache.
  - Anorexia, weight loss.
  - Restlessness: An akathisia-like state has been reported at initiation and termination of SSRIs.
  - Seizures: Rate of 0.2%, slightly lower than TCAs.

Serotonin syndrome is common when serotonergic drugs are used with MAOIs. SSRIs should not be used for at least 2 weeks before or after use of an MAOI.

- **Serotonin syndrome:** Caused by taking two drugs, both of which ↑ serotonin → too much serotonin in the brain. An example is triptans used with SSRIs. This is characterized by fever, diaphoresis, shivering, tachycardia, hypertension, delirium, and neuromuscular excitability (especially hyperreflexia and "electric jolt" limb movements), potentially → death.

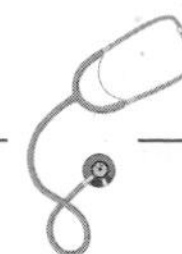

SSRIs can ↑ levels of warfarin, requiring ↑ monitoring when starting and stopping these medications.

Miscellaneous Antidepressants

SEROTONIN-NOREPINEPHRINE REUPTAKE INHIBITORS (SNRIS)

- **Venlafaxine (Effexor):**
  - Often used for depression, anxiety disorders like generalized anxiety disorder (GAD), and may have some use in attention deficit/hyperactivity disorder (ADHD).
  - Low drug interaction potential.
  - Extended release (XR form) allows for once-daily dosing.
  - Side effect profiles similar to SSRIs.
  - Can ↑ blood pressure (BP); do not use in patients with untreated or labile BP.
  - New form, **desvenlafaxine (Pristiq),** is the active metabolite of venlafaxine and is expensive.
- **Duloxetine (Cymbalta):**
  - Often used for people with **depression and neuropathic pain** or in fibromyalgia.
  - Side effects are similar to SSRIs, but more dry mouth and constipation relating to its norepinephrine effects.
  - There may be more liver side effects in patients with liver disease or heavy alcohol use.
  - Expensive.

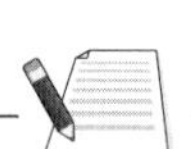

Bupropion can lower seizure threshold. Use with caution in patients with epilepsy and eating disorders.

NOREPINEPHRINE-DOPAMINE REUPTAKE INHIBITORS

- **Bupropion (Wellbutrin):**
  - Relative **lack of sexual side effects** as compared to the SSRIs.
  - Some efficacy in treatment of adult ADHD.
  - Side effects include ↑ risk of **seizures** and psychosis at high doses and ↑ anxiety in some.
  - Contraindicated in patients with seizure or active eating disorders and in those currently on an MAOI.

SEROTONIN RECEPTOR ANTAGONISTS AND AGONISTS

- **Trazodone (Desyrel)** and **Nefazodone (Serzone):**
  - Useful in treatment of refractory major depression, major depression with anxiety, and **insomnia** (secondary to its sedative effects).
  - They do not have the sexual side effects of SSRIs and do not affect rapid eye movement (REM) sleep.
  - Side effects include nausea, dizziness, orthostatic hypotension, cardiac arrhythmias, **sedation,** and **priapism** (especially with **trazodone**).
  - Nefazodone carries a **Black Box Warning** for rare but serious liver failure (1 per 250,000–300,000 people).

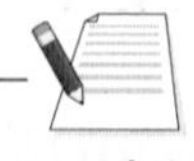

Trazodone causes priapism: t**RAZ**odone will **RAISE** the bone.

α_2-Adrenergic Receptor Antagonists

- **Mirtazapine (Remeron):**
  - Useful in the treatment of **refractory major depression,** especially in patients who need to gain weight.
  - Side effects include sedation, **weight gain,** dizziness, somnolence, tremor, dry mouth, constipation, and rare agranulocytosis.
  - No sexual side effects and few drug interactions.

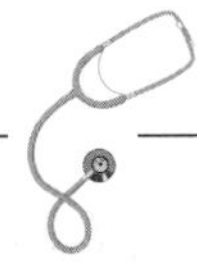

Remeron for depression in elderly—helps with sleep and appetite.

Heterocyclic Antidepressants: TCAs

- TCAs inhibit the reuptake of norepinephrine and serotonin, ↑ availability of monoamines in the synapse.
- Because of the long half-lives, most are dosed once daily.
- They are rarely used as first-line agents because they have a higher incidence of side effects, require greater monitoring of dosing, and can be **lethal in overdose.**

Tricyclic Antidepressants

- **Tertiary amines** (highly anticholinergic, more sedating, greater lethality in overdose):
  - **Amitriptyline (Elavil):** Useful in chronic pain, migraines, and insomnia.
  - **Imipramine (Tofranil):**
    - Has intramuscular form
    - Useful in enuresis and panic disorder
  - **Clomipramine (Anafranil):** Most serotonin specific, useful in treatment of OCD.
  - **Doxepin (Sinequan):**
    - Useful in treating chronic pain
    - Emerging use as a sleep aid in low doses
- **Secondary amines**—metabolites of tertiary amines (less anticholinergic, less sedating):
  - **Nortriptyline (Pamelor, Aventyl):**
    - Least likely to cause orthostatic hypotension
    - Useful therapeutic blood levels
    - Useful in treating chronic pain
  - **Desipramine (Norpramin):**
    - More activating; least sedating
    - Least anticholinergic

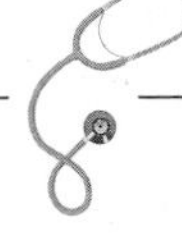

The mainstay of treatment for TCA overdose is IV sodium bicarbonate.

Tetracyclic Antidepressants

- **Amoxapine (Asendin):**
  - Metabolite of antipsychotic loxapine
  - May cause EPS and has similar side effect profile to typical antipsychotics
- **Maprotiline (Ludiomil):** Higher rates of seizure, arrhythmia, and fatality on overdose

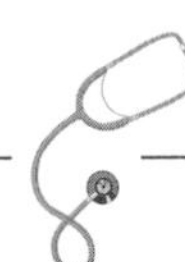

A 1-week supply of TCAs (as little as 1–2 g) can be lethal in overdose.

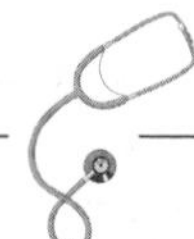

Major complications of TCAs—**3Cs:**
Cardiotoxicity
Convulsions
Coma

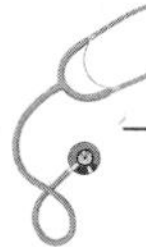

MAOIs are considered more effective in atypical depression characterized by hypersomnia, ↑ appetite, and ↑ sensitivity to interpersonal rejection.

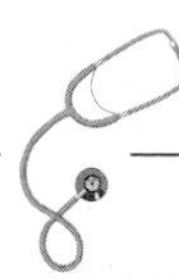

Selegiline (EMSAM patch) is an MAOI used to treat depression that does not require following the dietary restrictions when used in low dosages. However, decongestants, opiates (Demerol), and serotonergic drugs must still be avoided.

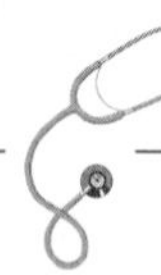

First step when suspecting serotonin syndrome: Discontinue medication. You can also try calcium channel blockers (oral nifedipine). If carefully monitored, you can try chlorpromazine or phentolamine.

Side Effects

- TCAs are *highly* protein bound and lipid soluble, and therefore can interact with other medications that have high protein binding.
- The side effects of TCAs are mostly due to their lack of specificity and interaction with other receptors.
- Antihistaminic properties: Sedation.
- Antiadrenergic properties (**cardiovascular** side effects): Orthostatic hypotension, dizziness, reflex tachycardia, arrhythmias, and electrocardiographic (ECG) changes (widening QRS, QT, and PR intervals). Avoid in patients with preexisting conduction abnormalities or recent MI.
- Antimuscarinic effects (also called anticholinergic): Dry mouth, constipation, urinary retention, blurred vision, tachycardia, exacerbation of narrow angle glaucoma.
- Weight gain.
- Lethal in overdose—must assess suicide risk! Agitation, tremors, ataxia, delirium, hypoventilation from central nervous system (CNS) depression, myoclonus, hyperreflexia, seizures, and coma are signs of overdose.
- Seizures: Occur at a rate of about 0.3%, more common at higher plasma levels and with clomipramine and tetracyclics.
- Serotonergic effects: Erectile/ejaculatory dysfunction in males, anorgasmia in females.

Monoamine Oxidase Inhibitors (MAOIs)

- MAOIs prevent the inactivation of biogenic amines such as *norepinephrine, serotonin, dopamine*, and *tyramine* (an intermediate in the conversion of tyrosine to norepinephrine).
- By irreversibly inhibiting the enzymes *MAO-A* and *-B*, MAOIs ↑ the number of neurotransmitters available in synapses.
- MAO-A preferentially deactivates serotonin, and MAO-B preferentially deactivates norepinephrine/epinephrine; *both* types also act on dopamine and tyramine.
- MAOIs are not used as first-line agents because of the ↑ safety and tolerability of newer agents. However, MAOIs are considered very effective for certain types of **refractory depression** and in refractory panic/anxiety disorder:
  - **Phenelzine (Nardil)**
  - **Tranylcypromine (Parnate)**
  - **Isocarboxazid (Marplan)**

Side Effects

- **Serotonin syndrome** occurs when **SSRIs** and **MAOIs** are taken together or if other drugs cause ↑ serotonin levels.
  - Initially characterized by lethargy, restlessness, confusion, flushing, diaphoresis, tremor, and myoclonic jerks.
  - May progress to hyperthermia, hypertonicity, rhabdomyolysis, renal failure, convulsions, coma, and death.
  - Wait at least 2 weeks before switching from SSRI to MAOI, and at least 5–6 weeks with fluoxetine.
- **Hypertensive crisis:** Risk when MAOIs are taken with tyramine-rich foods or sympathomimetics.

- Foods with tyramine (red wine, cheese, chicken liver, fava beans, cured meats) cause a buildup of stored catecholamines.
- In addition to markedly elevated BP, this is also characterized by headache, sweating, nausea and vomiting, photophobia, autonomic instability, chest pain, arrhythmias, and death.
- Orthostatic hypotension (most common).
- Drowsiness.
- Weight gain.
- Sexual dysfunction.
- Dry mouth.
- Sleep dysfunction.
- People with pyridoxine deficiency can have paresthesias, treated with B_6.
- Rarely, there is liver toxicity, seizures, and edema.
- Start low and go slow! (low doses that are ↑ slowly).

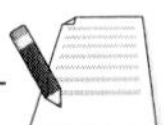

Wellbutrin (buproprion) can lower the seizure threshold, but it is *not* usually associated with sexual side effects of other antidepressants.

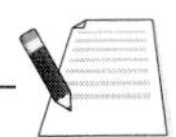

Dry mouth, retention, fatigue, and blurry vision are some of the side effects of TCAs. These can be attributed to the anticholinergic effects.

ANTIDEPRESSANT USE IN OTHER DISORDERS

- OCD: SSRIs (in high doses), TCAs (clomipramine)
- Panic disorder: SSRIs, TCAs (imipramine), MAOIs
- Eating disorders: SSRIs (in high doses), TCAs, and MAOIs
- Dysthymia: SSRIs
- Social phobia: SSRIs, TCAs, MAOIs
- GAD: SSRIs, SNRIs (venlafaxine), TCAs
- Posttraumatic stress disorder: SSRIs
- Irritable bowel syndrome: SSRIs, TCAs
- Enuresis: TCAs (imipramine)
- Neuropathic pain: TCAs (amitriptyline and nortriptyline), duloxetine
- Chronic pain: SSRIs, TCAs
- Fibromyalgia: SSRIs
- Migraine headaches: TCAs (amitriptyline), SSRIs
- Smoking cessation: Bupropion
- Premenstrual dysphoric disorder: SSRIs
- Depressive phase of manic depression: SSRIs
- Insomnia: Mirtazapine, TCAs (amitriptyline)

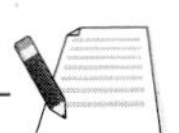

A patient on clozapine should have routine white blood cell (WBC) counts to monitor for agranulocytosis. These WBC counts should be performed weekly for the first 6 months of treatment and can ↓ in frequency thereafter.

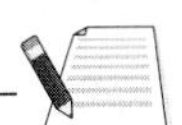

When prescribing lithium, it is important to monitor lithium, creatinine, and thyroid levels.

ANTIPSYCHOTICS

- Antipsychotics are used to treat psychotic disorders and psychotic symptoms associated with psychiatric and other medical illnesses.
  - *Typical* or *first-generation* antipsychotics, sometimes referred to as neuroleptics, are classified according to potency and treat psychosis by blocking dopamine (D2) receptors.
  - *Atypical* or *second-generation* antipsychotics (newer) antipsychotics block both dopamine (D2) and serotonin (2A) receptors.
- Most antipsychotics have a number of actions and receptor interactions in the brain that contribute to their varied efficacy and side effect profiles.
- Both typical and atypical antipsychotics have similar efficacies in treating the presence of *positive psychotic symptoms*, such as hallucinations and delusions.

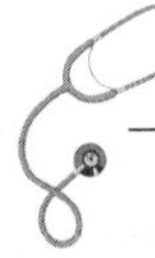

Warning about atypical antipsychotics: Although they are used to treat the symptoms of dementia and delirium, studies show an ↑ risk of all-cause mortality and stroke when using these agents in the elderly.

- Atypical antipsychotics may be more effective in treating *negative symptoms*, such as flattened affect and social withdrawal.
- Atypical antipsychotics had largely replaced typical antipsychotics in use due to their favorable side effect profile. However, evidence for metabolic syndrome, weight gain, and other previously underappreciated side effects, as well as the significant cost of these medications, means that currently both classes are first line.
- Each medication must be considered based on the patient and the side effect profile.

Typical Antipsychotics

All typical antipsychotics have similar efficacy, but vary in potency.

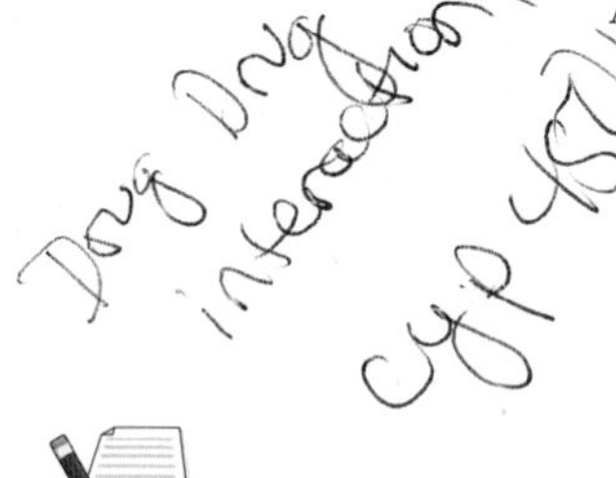

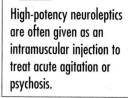

High-potency neuroleptics are often given as an intramuscular injection to treat acute agitation or psychosis.

Low-Potency, Typical Antipsychotics

- Have a lower affinity for dopamine receptors and therefore a higher dose is required. Remember, *potency* refers to the action on dopamine receptors, not the level of efficacy.
- There is a higher incidence of anticholinergic and antihistaminic side effects than high-potency traditional antipsychotics.
- Have a lower incidence of EPS and neuroleptic malignant syndrome.
- As a group, they have more lethality in overdose due to QTc prolongation and the potential for heart block and ventricular tachycardia.
- There is a rare risk for agranulocytosis, and they have a slightly higher seizure risk than higher-potency medications.
  - **Chlorpromazine (Thorazine):**
    - Commonly causes orthostatic hypotension
    - Can cause bluish skin discoloration
    - Can → photosensitivity
    - Can treat nausea and vomiting, as well as intractable hiccups
  - **Thioridazine (Mellaril):** Associated with retinitis pigmentosa

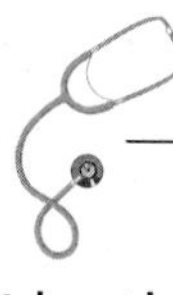

Haloperidol and fluphenazine are also available in long-acting, intramuscular forms (decanoate) that are useful if patients don't like taking oral medications. Risperidone (Consta) and paliperidone (Sustenna) also have long-acting injectibles, but they are more expensive.

Midpotency, Typical Antipsychotics

- Have midrange properties.
  - **Loxapine (Loxitane):**
    - Higher risk of seizure.
    - Metabolite is an antidepressant.
  - **Thiothixene (Navane):** Can cause ocular pigment changes
  - **Trifluoperazine (Stelazine):** Can reduce anxiety
  - **Perphenazine (Trilafon)**

High-Potency, Typical Antipsychotics

- Have greater affinity for dopamine receptors, and therefore a relatively low dose is needed to achieve effect.
- Cause less sedation, orthostatic hypotension, and anticholinergic effects.
- Greater risk for extrapyramidal symptoms and tardive dyskinesia.
  - **Haloperidol (Haldol):** Decanoate form available
  - **Fluphenazine (Prolixin):** Decanoate form available
  - **Pimozide (Orap):** Associated with heart block, ventricular tachycardia, and other cardiac effects

Side Effects

- The positive symptoms of schizophrenia are thought to be treated by action of medications in the mesolimbic dopamine pathway. The mesolimbic pathway includes the nucleus accumbens, the fornix, the amygdala, and the hippocampus.

- The negative symptoms of schizophrenia are thought to occur due to dopamine action in the mesocortical pathway.
- Extrapyramidal symptoms are thought to occur through the dopamine pathways in the nigrostriatum.
- ↑ prolactin is related to dopamine action in the tuberoinfundibular area.
- **Antidopaminergic effects:**
  - EPS:
    - *Parkinsonism*—bradykinesia, masklike face, cogwheel rigidity, pill-rolling tremor.
    - *Akathisia*—subjective anxiety and restlessness, objective fidgetiness. Patients may report a sensation of inability to sit still.
    - *Dystonia*—sustained painful contraction of muscles of neck *(torticollis)*, tongue, eyes *(oculogyric crisis)*. Life-threatening if they involve the airway or diaphragm.
  - **Hyperprolactinemia**—→ ↓ libido, galactorrhea, gynecomastia, impotence, amenorrhea, osteoporosis.
- **Anti-HAM effects:** Caused by actions on **H**istaminic, **A**drenergic, and **M**uscarinic receptors:
  - *Antihistaminic*—results in sedation, **weight gain**.
  - *Anti–α_1 adrenergic*—results in orthostatic hypotension, cardiac abnormalities, and sexual dysfunction.
  - *Antimuscarinic*—anticholinergic effects: results in dry mouth, tachycardia, urinary retention, blurry vision, constipation, and precipitation of narrow-angle glaucoma.
- **Tardive dyskinesia (TD):**
  - Choreoathetoid (writhing) movements of mouth and tongue (or other body parts) that may occur in patients who have used neuroleptics for > 6 months.
  - Most often occurs in older women.
  - Though 50% of cases will spontaneously remit, many cases may be *permanent*.
  - Treatment involves discontinuation of current antipsychotic if clinically possible and changing to a medication with less potential to cause tardive dyskinesia.
- Less common side effects include **neuroleptic malignant syndrome:**
  - Though rare, occurs most often in young males early in treatment with *both* atypical and typical antipsychotics.
  - It is a **medical emergency** and has a 20% mortality rate if left untreated.
  - It is characterized by:
    - **F**ever (most common presenting symptom)
    - **A**utonomic instability (tachycardia, labile hypertension, diaphoresis)
    - **L**eukocytosis
    - **T**remor
    - **E**levated creatine phosphokinase (CPK)
    - **R**igidity (*lead pipe* rigidity is considered almost universal)
    - **E**xcessive sweating (diaphoresis)
    - **D**elirium
  - **Treatment** involves discontinuation of current medications and administration of supportive medical care (hydration, cooling, etc.).

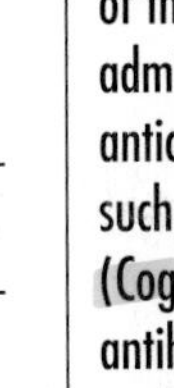

Treatment of extrapyramidal symptoms includes reducing the dose of the antipsychotic and administering an anticholinergic medication such as benztropine (Cogentin), an antihistaminergic medication such as diphenhydramine (Benadryl), or an antiparkinsonian medication such as amantadine (Symmetrel).

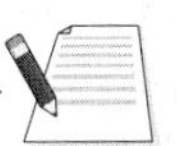

Clozapine, the first atypical antipsychotic, is less likely to cause tardive dyskinesia.

- Sodium dantrolene, bromocriptine, and amantadine are infrequently used because of their own side effects and unclear efficacy.
- This is *not* an allergic reaction.
- Patient is not prevented from restarting the same neuroleptic at a later time.
- Elevated liver enzymes, jaundice.
- **Ophthalmologic** problems (irreversible retinal pigmentation with high doses of thioridazine, deposits in lens and cornea with chlorpromazine).
- **Dermatologic** problems, including rashes and photosensitivity (blue-gray skin discoloration with chlorpromazine).
- **Seizures:** Antipsychotics lower seizure thresholds. Low-potency antipsychotics are more likely to cause seizures than high potency.

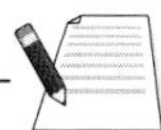

There is a roughly 1% chance of developing tardive dyskinesia for each year on a typical antipsychotic.

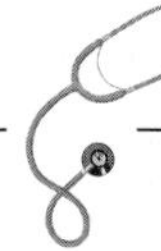

Onset of Neuroleptic Side Effects

Acute dystonia: Hours to days
EPS/Akathisia: Days to months
TD: Months to years
Abnormal Involuntary Movement Scale (AIMS) can be used to quantify and monitor for tardive dyskinesia.

Ms. Brown is a 31-year-old, overweight woman who presents to your outpatient clinic following discharge from an inpatient psychiatry unit. Police found her in a local shopping mall, talking to herself and telling passersby that the devil had "stolen her soul." She appeared disheveled and scared. During the hospitalization, she was diagnosed with schizophrenia, and olanzapine was prescribed and titrated to 30 mg at bedtime for delusional thinking and disorganized behavior. She has been living with her parents, and her hygiene and self-care have improved. Although Ms. Brown reports occasional auditory hallucinations telling her that her parents do not like her, she recognizes that the voices are not real and is not distressed by them. Ms. Brown has become involved in a vocational skills program and hopes to work at a local supermarket. However, during her last appointment with her primary care doctor, she was told she had an elevated fasting glucose of 115, had gained 12 pounds in the past 3 months, her waist circumference was 36 inches, and her triglycerides were found to be 180. Her blood pressure was normal, and she reported a family history of diabetes and high blood pressure.

What is the next step?

Given that Ms. Brown has had an adequate partial response to pharmacological treatment, she should continue to be treated with an antipsychotic. However, her recent laboratory results are suggestive of metabolic syndrome, and thus she is at an ↑ risk for cardiovascular disease. While this patient has responded well to olanzapine, this medication along with other atypical antipsychotics, have been associated with ↑ weight gain and impaired glucose metabolism. It is unclear if Ms. Brown's laboratory test results were abnormal prior to starting olanzapine or are elevated secondary to treatment, possibly a combination of both. In treating Ms. Brown, first steps include recommending lifestyle modifications and close monitoring of her weight, blood sugar levels, lipids, and waist circumference while collaborating closely with her primary care physician. If a change in her antipsychotic medication is warranted after weighing the risks and benefits of altering her treatment, other atypical antipsychotics such as ziprasidone or aripiprazole (less associated with weight gain) or typical antipsychotics might be considered; these medications would be cross-tapered. When choosing medications, consideration must be given to history of response, tolerability, side effect profile, and cost.

Atypical Antipsychotics

- Atypical antipsychotics block both dopamine and serotonin receptors and are associated with different side effects than traditional antipsychotics.
- In particular, they are less likely to cause EPS, tardive dyskinesia, or neuroleptic malignant syndrome.
- They may be more effective in treating **negative symptoms** of schizophrenia than traditional antipsychotics.
- Atypical antipsychotics are also used to treat acute mania, bipolar disorder, and as adjunctive medications in unipolar depression.
- They are sometimes used for personality disorders and certain psychiatric disorders in childhood.
  - **Clozapine (Clozaril):**
    - Less likely to cause tardive dyskinesia.
    - Only antipsychotic shown to be *more* efficacious.
    - Associated with tachycardia and hypersalivation.
    - More anticholinergic side effects than other atypical or high-potency typicals.
    - Myocarditis can develop.
    - There is a 1–2% incidence of **agranulocytosis** and 2–5% incidence of **seizures.**
    - You must stop clozapine if the *absolute neutrophil count* drops below 1500/µL.
    - Clozapine is the only antipsychotic shown to ↓ **the risk of suicide.**
  - **Risperidone (Risperdal):**
    - Can cause ↑ prolactin
    - Some orthostatic hypotension and reflex tachycardia
    - Has long-acting injectable form called Consta
  - **Quetiapine (Seroquel):** Common side effects include sedation and orthostatic hypotension.
  - **Olanzapine (Zyprexa):** Common side effect is weight gain.
  - **Ziprasidone (Geodon):** Less likely to cause weight gain.
  - **Aripiprazole (Abilify):**
    - Unique mechanism of partial D2 agonism
    - Can be more activating (akathisia) and less sedating
    - Less potential for weight gain
- Newer, expensive medications:
  - **Paliperidone (Invega):**
    - Metabolite of risperidone
    - Long-acting injectable form (Sustenna)
  - **Asenapine (Saphris)**
  - **Iloperidone (Fanapt)**

Side Effects

- **Metabolic syndrome.**
- This must be monitored with baseline weight, waist circumference (measured at iliac crest), blood pressure, fasting glucose, and fasting lipids (triglycerides).
- Some anti-HAM effects (antihistaminic, antiadrenergic, and antimuscarinic).
- **Weight gain.**
- Hyperlipidemia.
- Hyperglycemia—rarely, **diabetic ketoacidosis** has been reported.

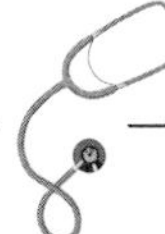

Thirty percent of treatment-resistant psychosis will respond to clozapine.

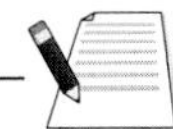

Haldol has extrapyramidal side effects such as tardive dyskinesia, but does not typically → agranulocytosis, which is associated with medications such as clozapine.

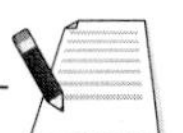

Tacrine and donepezil, Alzheimer medications, work by reversible inhibition of aceytlcholine esterase.

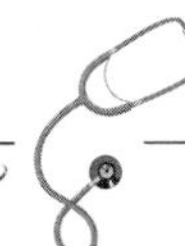

Quetiapine, olanzapine, aripiprazole, risperidone, and ziprasidone have FDA approval for treatment of mania.

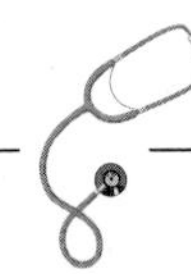

Patients on clozapine must have weekly blood draws for the first 6 months to check absolute neutrophil count and WBC counts because this medication can cause agranulocytosis. With time, the frequency of blood draws ↓.

- Liver function—monitor yearly for elevation in liver function tests and ammonia.
- QTc prolongation.

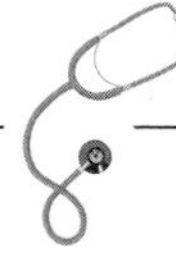

Antipsychotics may be used as adjuncts to mood stabilizers early in the course of a manic episode.

MOOD STABILIZERS

- Mood stabilizers are used to treat **acute mania** and to help **prevent relapses** of manic episodes in bipolar disorder and schizoaffective disorder. Less commonly, they may be used for:
  - Potentiation of antidepressants in patients with major depression refractory to monotherapy
  - Potentiation of antipsychotics in patients with schizophrenia
  - Enhancement of abstinence in treatment of alcoholism
  - Treatment of aggression and impulsivity (dementia, intoxication, mental retardation, personality disorders, general medical conditions
- Mood stabilizers include lithium and anticonvulsants, most commonly valproic acid, lamotrigine, and carbamazepine.

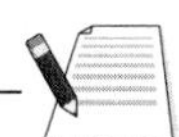

Lithium is the only mood stabilizer shown to ↓ **suicidality.**

Lithium

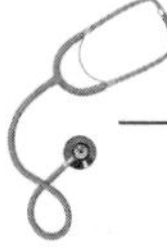

Blood levels are useful for lithium, valproic acid, carbamazepine, and clozapine.

- Lithium is the drug of choice in acute mania and as prophylaxis for both manic and depressive episodes in bipolar and schizoaffective disorders.
- It is also used in cyclothymia and unipolar depression.
- Lithium is metabolized by the kidney, and so you have to adjust the dose and monitor levels closely if patient has renal dysfunction.
- Prior to initiating, patients should have an ECG, basic chemistries, thyroid function tests, a complete blood count, and a pregnancy test.
- Onset of action takes 5–7 days.
- Blood levels correlate with clinical efficacy and should be checked after 5 days, and then every 2–3 days until therapeutic.
- The major drawback of lithium is its high incidence of side effects and very narrow therapeutic index:
  - Therapeutic range: 0.6 to 1.2 (Individual patients can become toxic even within this range.)
  - Toxic: > 1.5
  - Lethal: > 2.0

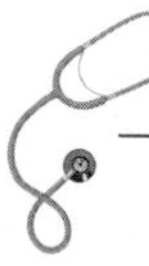

Think twice before prescribing ibuprofen to a patient on lithium.

Side Effects

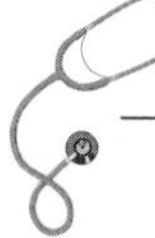

Factors that affect Li+ levels:

- NSAIDs (↓)
- Aspirin
- Dehydration (↑)
- Salt deprivation (↑)
- Sweating (salt loss) (↑)
- Impaired renal function (↑)
- Diuretics, especially thiazides

- Toxic levels of lithium cause altered mental status, coarse tremors, convulsions, and death.
- Clinicians need to regularly monitor blood levels of lithium, thyroid function (thyroid-stimulating hormone), and kidney function.
- Fine tremor.
- Nephrogenic diabetes insipidus.
- GI disturbance.
- Weight gain.
- Sedation.
- Thyroid enlargement, hypothyroidism.
- ECG changes.
- Benign leukocytosis.
- Lithium can cause **Ebstein's anomaly,** a cardiac defect in babies born to mothers taking lithium.

ANTICONVULSANTS

Carbamazepine (Tegretol)

- Especially useful in treating *mixed* episodes and *rapid-cycling* bipolar disorder, and less effective for the depressed phase.
- Also used in the management of trigeminal neuralgia.
- Acts by blocking sodium channels and inhibiting action potentials.
- Onset of action is 5–7 days.
- Complete blood count (CBC) and liver function tests (LFTs) must be obtained before initiating treatment and monitored regularly.

> The side effect of leukocytosis can sometimes be advantageous when combined with other medications that ↓ WBC count (eg, clozapine).

Side Effects

- The most common side effects are GI and CNS (drowsiness, ataxia, sedation, confusion).
- Possible skin rash **(Stevens-Johnson Syndrome).**
- Leukopenia, hyponatremia, aplastic anemia, thrombocytopenia, and agranulocytosis.
- Elevation of liver enzymes, causing hepatitis.
- **Teratogenic** effects when used during pregnancy (neural tube defects).
- It also has significant drug interactions with many drugs metabolized by the cytochrome P450 pathway, including inducing its own metabolism through *autoinduction*, requiring increasing dosages.
- Toxicity: Confusion, stupor, motor restlessness, ataxia, tremor, nystagmus, twitching, and vomiting.

Valproic Acid (Depakote and Depakene)

- Useful in treating mixed episodes of bipolar disorder as well as rapid cycling.
- Monitoring of LFTs and CBC is necessary.
- Drug levels are usually checked after 3–5 days. The normal range is 50–150 micrograms/mL.
- **Lamotrigine (Lamictal):**
  - Efficacy for **bipolar depression,** though little efficacy for acute mania or prevention of mania.
  - Works on sodium channels that modulate glutamate and aspartate.
  - Most common side effects are dizziness, sedation, headaches, and ataxia.
  - The most serious side effect is **Stevens-Johnson syndrome** (a life-threatening rash involving skin and mucous membranes) in 10%. This is most likely in the first 4–6 weeks, but this is minimized by starting with low doses and increasing them *slowly.*
  - Valproate will ↑ lamotrigine levels, and lamotrigine will ↓ valproate levels.
- **Oxcarbazepine (Trileptal):**
  - As effective in mood disorders as carbamazepine, but better tolerated
  - Less risk of rash and hepatic toxicity
- **Gabapentin (Neurontin):**
  - Often used adjunctively to help with anxiety, sleep
  - Little efficacy in bipolar disorder
- **Pregabalin (Lyrica):**
  - Used in generalized anxiety disorder and fibromyalgia
  - Little efficacy in bipolar disorder

- **Tiagabine (Gabitril):** May be helpful with anxiety
- **Topiramate (Topamax):**
  - Helpful with impulse control disorder and anxiety
  - Beneficial side effect is **weight loss**
  - Can cause hypochloremic, non–anion gap metabolic acidosis and kidney stones
  - The most limiting side effect is **cognitive slowing**

SIDE EFFECTS

- GI side effects
- Weight gain
- Sedation
- Alopecia
- Pancreatitis
- **Hepatotoxicity** or benign aminotransferase elevations
- ↑ ammonia
- Thrombocytopenia
- **Teratogenic** effects during pregnancy (neural tube defects)

ANXIOLYTICS/HYPNOTICS

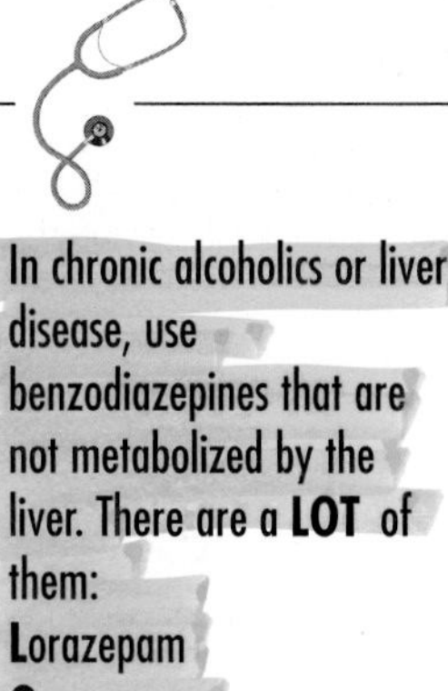

In chronic alcoholics or liver disease, use benzodiazepines that are not metabolized by the liver. There are a **LOT** of them:
Lorazepam
Oxazepam
Temazepam

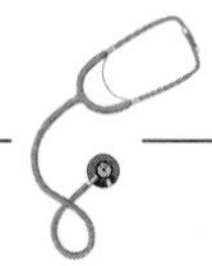

BDZs can be lethal when mixed with alcohol. Respiratory depression causes death.

- Anxiolytics, including benzodiazepines, barbiturates, and buspirone, are the most widely prescribed psychotropic medications.
- Common indications for anxiolytics/hypnotics include:
  - Anxiety disorders
  - Muscle spasm
  - Seizures
  - Sleep disorders
  - Alcohol withdrawal
  - Anesthesia induction

Benzodiazepines (BDZs)

- Benzodiazepines work by potentiating the effects of gamma-aminobutyric acid (GABA).
- They do reduce anxiety.
- Many patients become dependent on these medications and require increasing amounts for the same clinical effect.
- Potential for abuse.
- Choice of benzodiazepine is based on time to onset of action, duration of action, and method of metabolism.
- Relatively safer in overdose than barbiturates.

Long Acting (Half-life: > 20 hours)
- **Diazepam (Valium):**
  - Rapid onset.
  - Used during detoxification from alcohol or sedative-hypnotic-anxiolytics and for seizures.
  - Less commonly prescribed to treat anxiety than previously.
- **Clonazepam (Klonopin):**
  - Treatment of anxiety, including panic attacks.
  - Avoid with renal dysfunction; longer half-life allows for once daily dosing.

Abrupt withdrawal can cause seizures and confusion

Intermediate Acting (Half-life: 6–20 Hours)

- **Alprazolam (Xanax):**
  - Treatment of anxiety, including panic attacks
  - Short onset of action → euphoria, high abuse potential
- **Lorazepam (Ativan):**
  - Treatment of panic attacks; alcohol and sedative-hypnotic-anxiolytic detoxification; agitation
  - Not metabolized by liver
- **Oxazepam (Serax):**
  - Alcohol and sedative-hypnotic-anxiolytic detoxification
  - Not metabolized by liver
- **Temazepam (Restoril):**
  - Decreasingly used for treatment of insomnia due to dependence
  - Not metabolized by liver

Short Acting (Half-life: < 6 hours)

- **Triazolam (Halcion):**
  - Treatment of insomnia
  - Primarily used in medical and surgical settings
- **Midazolam (Versed):** Primarily used in medical and surgical settings

> For benzodiazepine overdose, **flumazenil** is used to reverse the effects of benzodiazepine receptor agonists. However, be careful not to induce withdrawal too quickly—this can be life threatening.

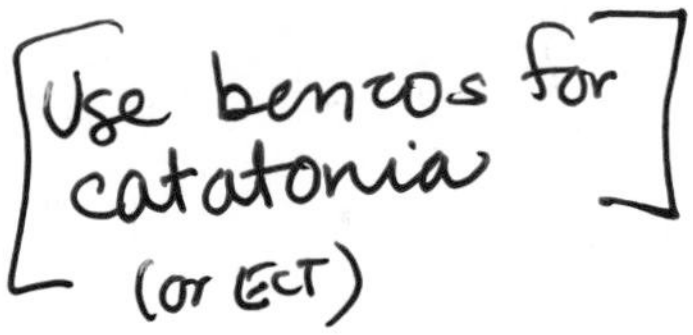
Use benzos for catatonia
(or ECT)

Side Effects

- Drowsiness
- Impairment of intellectual function
- Reduced motor coordination (careful in elderly)
- Anterograde amnesia
- Withdrawal can be life threatening and causes seizures
- Toxicity: Respiratory depression in overdose, especially when combined with alcohol

Non-Benzodiazepine Hypnotics

- **Zolpidem (Ambien)/zaleplon(Sonata)/eszopiclone (Lunesta):**
  - These medications work by selective receptor binding to benzodiazepine receptor 1, which is responsible for sedation.
  - These medications are used for short-term treatment of insomnia.
  - Less tolerance/dependence occurs with prolonged use (but still can occur).
  - Zaleplon has a shorter half-life than zolpidem, which has a shorter half-life than eszopiclone.
  - Reports of anterograde amnesia, hallucinations, sleepwalking, and other behaviors may limit their tolerability, as well as the more commonly reported GI side effects.
- **Diphenhydramine (Benadryl):**
  - An antihistamine.
  - Side effects include sedation, dry mouth, constipation, urinary retention, and blurry vision.
- **Chloral hydrate (Noctec, Somnote):**
  - Not commonly prescribed due to tolerance and dependence
  - Lethal in overdose, causing hepatic and liver failure
- **Ramelteon (Rozerem):**
  - Selective melatonin MT1 and MT2 agonist
  - No tolerance or dependence

Non-Benzodiazepine Anxiolytics

- **Buspirone (BuSpar):**
  - The anxiolytic action is at 5HT-1A receptor (partial agonist).
  - It has a slower onset of action than BDZ (takes 1–2 weeks for effect).
  - Not considered as effective as other options, and so it is often used in combination with another agent (eg, an SSRI), for treatment of anxiety.
  - It does not potentiate the CNS depression of alcohol (useful in alcoholics), and has a low potential for abuse/addiction.
- **Hydroxyzine (Atarax):**
  - An antihistamine.
  - Side effects include sedation, dry mouth, constipation, urinary retention, and blurry vision.
  - Useful for patients who want quick-acting, short-term medication, but who cannot take benzodiazepines for various reasons.
- **Barbiturates** (eg, **butalbitol, phenobarbitol, amobarbitol, pentobarbitol**): Rarely used now because of the lethality of overdose and side effect profile.
- **Propranolol:**
  - Beta blocker.
  - Useful in treating the autonomic effects of panic attacks or performance anxiety, such as palpitations, sweating, and tachycardia.
  - It can also be used to treat akathisia (side effect of typical antipsychotics).

PSYCHOSTIMULANTS

Used in ADHD and in treatment refractory depression.

- **Dextroamphetamine and amphetamines (Dexedrine, Adderall):**
  - Dextroamphetamine is the D-isomer of amphetamine.
  - Adderall is Schedule II, which means Rx in triplicate and high potential for **abuse.**
  - Monitor BP and watch for weight loss, insomnia.
- **Methylphenidate (Ritalin, Concerta):**
  - CNS stimulant, similar to amphetamine.
  - Schedule II, which means Rx in triplicate and high potential for abuse.
  - Watch for leukopenia, anemia, ↑ LFTs—monitor labs.
  - Monitor BP and watch for weight loss, insomnia.
- **Atomoxetine (Strattera):**
  - Presynaptic norepinephrine transporter inhibitor
  - Less appetite suppression and insomnia
  - Rare liver toxicity, possible ↑ SI in children/adolescents
- **Modafanil (Provigil):** Used in narcolepsy

COGNITIVE ENHANCERS

Used in dementia.

loss of cholinergic neurons in Alzheimer's

ACETYLCHOLINESTERASE INHIBITORS

- **Donepezil (Aricept):**
  - Once daily dosing
  - Some GI effects
  - Mild to moderate dementia
- **Galantamine (Reminyl)**
- **Rivastigmine (Excelon):** Has a patch, less side effects
- **Tacrine (Cognex)**
- **Memantine (Namenda):**
  - Moderate to severe dementia
  - Better together with acetylcholinesterase inhibitor

SUMMARY OF MEDICATIONS THAT MAY CAUSE PSYCHIATRIC SYMPTOMS

Psychosis

May be caused by sympathomimetics, analgesics, antibiotics (such as isoniazid), anticholinergics, anticonvulsants, antihistamines, corticosteroids, and anti-parkinsonian agents.

Agitation/Confusion/Delirium

May be caused by antipsychotics, antidepressants, antiarrhythmics, antineoplastics, corticosteroids, cardiac glycosides, nonsteroidal anti-inflammatories (NSAIDs), antiasthmatics, antibiotics, antihypertensives, antiparkinsonian agents, thyroid hormones.

Depression

May be caused by antihypertensives, antiparkinsonian agents, corticosteroids, calcium channel blockers, NSAIDs, antibiotics, peptic ulcer drugs.

Anxiety

May be caused by sympathomimetics, antiasthmatics, antiparkinsonian agents, hypoglycemic, NSAIDs, thyroid hormones.

Sedation/Poor Concentration

May be caused by antianxiety agents/hypnotics, anticholinergics, antibiotics, antihistamines.

Selected Medications

- **Procainamide, quinidine:** Confusion, delirium
- **Albuterol:** Anxiety, confusion
- **Isoniazid:** Psychosis
- **Tetracycline:** Depression
- **Nifedipine, verapamil:** Depression
- **Cimetidine:** Depression, psychosis
- **Steroids:** Aggressiveness/agitation, hypomania, anxiety, psychosis

OTHER TREATMENTS

Electroconvulsive Therapy (ECT)

Patients are given general anesthesia (often methohexital), and muscle relaxants (often succinylcholine), and then a generalized tonic-clonic seizure is induced using unilateral or bilateral electrodes. Effectiveness is based on the length of *postictal suppression* and other factors, not on seizure duration. This is an effective treatment for depression especially with psychotic features, acute mania, and catatonia. It is often used in patients who cannot tolerate medications or who have failed other treatments. ECT is discontinued after symptomatic improvement, typically 8–12 sessions given three times weekly, and monthly *maintenance ECT* is often used to prevent relapse of symptoms. The most common side effect is muscle soreness, headaches, amnesia, and confusion. Bilateral electrode placements ↓ the number of treatments needed, but ↑ memory impairment and confusion.

Deep Brain Stimulation (DBS)

Deep brain stimulation (DBS) is a surgical treatment involving the implantation of a medical device that sends electrical impulses to specific parts of the brain. DBS in select brain regions has provided benefits for chronic pain, Parkinson disease, tremor, and dystonia. Its underlying principles and mechanisms are still not clear. DBS directly changes brain activity in a controlled manner and its effects are reversible (unlike those of lesioning techniques). DBS has been used to treat various affective disorders, including major depression. While DBS has proven helpful for some patients, there is potential for serious complications and side effects.

Repetitive Transcranial Magnetic Stimulation (rTMS)

rTMS is a noninvasive method to excite neurons in the brain. Weak electric currents are induced in the tissue by rapidly changing magnetic fields, a process called electromagnetic induction. This way, brain activity can be triggered with minimal discomfort. rTMS and can produce longer lasting changes than nonrepetitive stimulation. Numerous small-scale studies have shown it could be a treatment tool for some psychiatric conditions (eg, major depression, auditory hallucinations). Most studies show modest effects at best. Side effects include rare seizure and discomfort at the delivery site.

Light Therapy

Light therapy or phototherapy consists of exposure to daylight or to specific wavelengths of light using lasers, light-emitting diodes, fluorescent lamps, dichroic lamps or very bright, full-spectrum light, for a prescribed amount of time and, in some cases, at a specific time of day. Bright light to the eyes treats seasonal affective disorder, with some support for its use also with nonseasonal psychiatric disorders.

HIGH-YIELD FACTS IN

Forensic Psychiatry

Forensic psychiatry is a medical subspecialty that includes the many areas in which psychiatry is applied to legal issues. Forensic psychiatrists often conduct evaluations requested by the court or attorneys.

While some forensic psychiatrists may specialize exclusively in legal issues, almost all psychiatrists may have to work within one of the many areas in which the mental health and legal system overlap. These areas include the following:

- Risk assessment
- Criminal responsibility
- Competence/decisional capacity
- Child custody and visitation
- Psychic injury
- Mental disability
- Malpractice
- Involuntary treatment
- Correctional psychiatry

Legal issues are considered **criminal** in nature if someone is being charged with a crime. **Civil** cases involve other kinds of rights and may result in monetary awards. The specific laws pertaining to the various topics discussed in this chapter often vary state by state.

STANDARD OF CARE AND MALPRACTICE

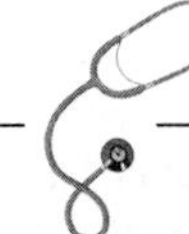

A wrong prediction or a bad outcome is not necessarily proof of bad doctoring.

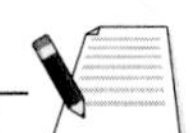

4 D's of malpractice: **D**eviation (neglect) from **D**uty that was the **D**irect cause of **D**amage

- The **standard of care** in psychiatry is generally defined as the skill level and knowledge base of the average, prudent psychiatrist in a given community.
- **Negligence** is practicing below the standard of care.
- **Malpractice** is the act of being negligent as a doctor.
- The following four conditions must be proven by a preponderance of the evidence to sustain a claim of malpractice:
  1. The physician had a duty of care (psychiatrist-patient relationship).
  2. The physician breached his or her duty by practice that did not meet the standard of care (negligence).
  3. The patient was harmed.
  4. The harm was directly caused by the physician's negligence.
- If a malpractice case is successful, the patient can receive **compensatory damages** (reimbursement for medical expenses, lost salary, or physical suffering) and **punitive damages** (money awarded to "punish" the doctor).

CONFIDENTIALITY

All information regarding a doctor-patient relationship should be held confidential, when otherwise exempted by statute, such as:

- When sharing relevant information with other staff members who are also treating the patient.
- If subpoenaed—physician must supply all requested information.

- If child abuse is suspected—obligated to report to the proper authorities.
- If a patient is suicidal—physician may need to admit the patient, with or without the patient's consent, and share information with the hospital staff.

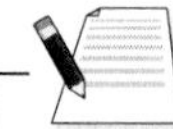

The obligation of a physician to report patients who are potentially harmful to others is called the *Tarasoff duty*, based on a landmark legal case.

DECISION MAKING

Informed Consent

- Process by which patients knowingly and voluntarily agree to a treatment or procedure.
- In order to make informed decisions, patients must know the purpose of the treatment, alternative treatments, and the potential risks and benefits of undergoing and of refusing the treatment.
- The patient should have the opportunity to ask questions.
- Situations that do not require informed consent:
  - Lifesaving medical emergency
  - Prevention of suicidal or homicidal behavior
  - Unemancipated minors receiving obstetric care, sexually transmitted disease (STD) treatment, or substance abuse treatment

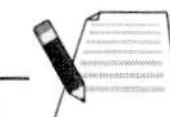

Elements of informed consent **(4 R's):**
Reason for treatment
Risks and benefits
Reasonable alternatives
Refused treatment consequences

Emancipated Minors

- Considered competent to give consent for all medical care without parental input or consent
- Minors are considered emancipated if they are:
  - Self-supporting
  - In the military
  - Married
  - Have children

Emancipated minors do not need parental consent to make medical decisions.

Decisional Capacity

Competence and *capacity* are terms that refer to a patient's ability to make informed treatment decisions.

- *Capacity* is a clinical term and may be assessed by physicians.
- *Competence* is a legal term and can be decided only by a judge.
- Decisional capacity is *task specific* and can fluctuate over time.
- In order for a patient to have decisional capacity, he or she must be able to:
  - Understand the relevant information regarding treatment (purpose, risks, benefits).
  - Appreciate the appropriate weight and impact of the decision.
  - Logically manipulate the information to make a decision.
  - Communicate a choice or preference.
- Criteria for determining capacity may be more stringent if the consequences of a patient's decision are very serious.

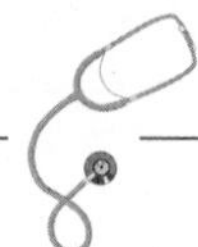

As a result of the *Tarasoff* case, when a physician is treating a patient who may physically harm another individual(s), the physician is obligated to warn potential victims about the impending threat.

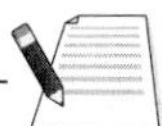

Doctors are required to report child abuse, but lawyers are not.

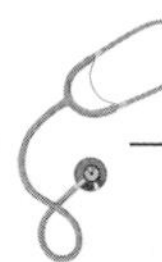

If a child presents to the emergency department with various bruises and numerous prior emergency room visits, your next step is to contact appropriate authorities.

Guardians and Conservators

- May be appointed by a judge to make treatment decisions for incompetent patients.
- Should make decisions by substituted judgment (what the patient would most likely have expressed were the patient competent).
- Several laws have been implemented to deal with the mentally ill. The **M'Naghten test** is important in cases involving an insanity plea because it addresses whether the patient comprehends the measure and quality of his or her actions and whether he or she knows that his or her actions are wrong. It is also important to establish whether or not a person is competent in understanding the risks and benefits of the medical treatment being offered. Involuntary admission is sometimes required if the patient appears to be a danger to his or her self and others.

ADMISSION TO A PSYCHIATRIC HOSPITAL

The two main categories of admission to a psychiatric hospital are voluntary and involuntary.

- **Voluntary:**
  - Patient requests or agrees to be admitted to the psychiatric ward.
  - Voluntary patients may not have the right to be discharged immediately upon request.
  - Patient must be competent to be admitted inpatient as a voluntary patient.
- **Involuntary:**
  - Patient must be found to be harmful to self or others or unable to provide for his/her basic needs.
  - Involuntary patients have legal rights to a trial to challenge their hospitalization.
  - Involuntary patients do not automatically lose the right to refuse treatment, including the involuntary administration of medication.
  - Involuntary commitment is supported by legal principles of **police power** (protecting citizens from each other) and **parens patriae** (protecting citizens who can't care for themselves).

DISABILITY

- **Mental impairment:** Loss, loss of use, or derangement of a mental function
- **Mental disability:** Alteration of an individual's capacity to meet personal, social, or occupational demands due to a mental impairment
- To assess whether an impairment is also a disability, consider four categories:
  - Activities of daily living
  - Social functioning
  - Concentration, persistence, and pace
  - Deterioration or decomposition in work settings

COMPETENCE TO STAND TRAIL

- *Competence* is a legal term for the capacity to understand, rationally manipulate, and apply information to make a reasoned decision on a specific issue. This definition varies by state.
- The 6th and 14th Amendments to the Constitution require that someone cannot be tried if they are not mentally competent to stand trial.
- This was established by the legal case *Dusky vs. United States* in 1960.
- If a defendant has significant mental health problems or behaves irrationally in court, his competency to stand trial should be considered.
- Competence may vary over time.
- To stand trial, a defendant must:
  - Understand the charges against him or her.
  - Be familiar with the courtroom personnel.
  - Have the ability to work with an attorney and participate in his or her trial.
  - Understand possible consequences.

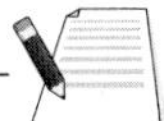

6th Amendment: Right to counsel and to confront witnesses

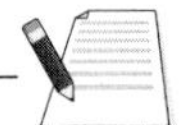

14th Amendment: Right to due process of law

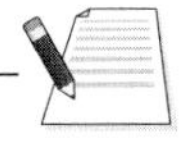

The fact that someone is mentally ill doesn't mean they can't be competent to stand trial.

NOT GUILTY BY REASON OF INSANITY (NGRI)

- Conviction of a crime requires both an "evil deed" *(actus reus)* and "evil intent" *(mens rea).*
- **Insanity** is a legal term, and its definition varies by state (see Table 18-1).
- If someone is declared legally insane, they are not criminally responsible for their act.
- Some states have a ruling of Guilty but Mentally Ill (GBMI) instead of NGRI or no criminal insanity defense at all.
- NGRI is used in 1% of criminal cases.
- It is successful in 2.5% of cases that use it.
- NGRI acquitees often spend the same amount of time or more as involuntary psychiatric patients than they would have in prison if they were found guilty.

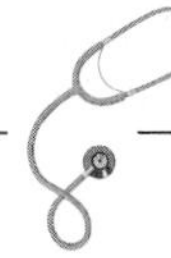

After John Hinckley received NGRI for an assignation attempt on President Reagan, there was public outcry against lenient NGRI standards, contributing to the Insanity Defense Reform Act of 1983.

TABLE 18-1. Insanity Defense Standards

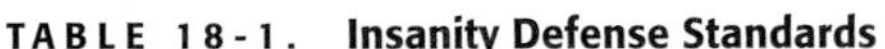

STANDARD	DEFINITION
M'Naghten	▪ Person does not understand what he was doing *or* its wrongfulness. ▪ Most stringent test.
American Law Institute (ALI) Model Penal Code	Person could not appreciate right from wrong *or* could not control actions (also known as the "irresistible impulse" test).
Durham	▪ The person's criminal act has resulted from mental illness. ▪ Most lenient test and is rarely used.

TABLE 18-2. Correlations of Mental Illness and Violence Toward Self/Others

Mental Illness	↑ risk of violence
Schizophrenia	Controversial, ranges from 2×–5×
Depression	~5×
Bipolar Disorder	~5×
Alcohol Abuse/Dependence	~12×
Other Substance Abuse/Dependence	~16×

RISK ASSESSMENT

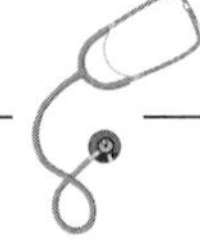

The most important factor in assessing a patient's risk of violence is the individual's history of violence.

- **Violence risk factors** (see Table 18-2):
  - History of violence
  - Specific threat with a plan
  - History of impulsivity
  - Psychiatric diagnosis
  - Substance abuse
- **Predicting dangerousness:**
  - Short-term easier than long-term
  - High false positives because of low base rates (most people are not violent)

OTHER AREAS OF FORENSIC PSYCHIATRY

Expert Witness Standards

- *Frye* (1923): Evidence must be generally accepted by the appropriate scientific community.
- *Daubert* (1993): Judge decides if evidence is based on relevant and reliable science.

Malingering

- Feigning or exaggerating symptoms for "secondary gain," including:
  - Financial gain (injury law suit)
  - Avoiding school, work, or other responsibilities
  - Obtaining medications of abuse (opioids, benzodiazepines)
  - Avoiding legal consequences
- Signs for detecting malingering:
  - Atypical presentation
  - "Textbook" description of the illness
  - History of working in the medical field
  - Symptoms that are present only when the patient knows he/she is being observed
  - History of substance abuse or antisocial personality disorder

Child and Family Law

Evaluations that a child forensic psychiatrist may be needed for include:

- Child custody
- Termination of parental rights
- Child abuse or neglect

Correctional Psychiatry

- With the closing of state psychiatric hospitals (ie, deinstutionalization), many persons with mental illness have moved to correctional institutions.
- Psychiatrists who practice in jails and prisons must balance treating inmates as patients and maintaining safety in the institution.
- Issues of **confidentiality** and **violence** are key.

A 65-year-old African-American male with insulin-dependent diabetes mellitus and severe major depressive disorder was admitted to the intensive care unit for treatment of diabetic ketoacidosis. The internal medicine team calls your psychiatry consult-liaison service to evaluate the patient for depression and provide treatment recommendations.

When you meet the patient, he is disoriented, confused, and has a waxing and waning level of consciousness. His mini-mental status exam (MMSE) score is 18/30. You identify that the patient is likely delirious, and you are unable to obtain any useful historical information. After interviewing the patient's daughter by phone, you learn that he has had progressively worsening depressive symptoms over the past year. The patient's wife passed away 2 years ago, and he has told family members that he can no longer live without her. His daughter recently found him in the garage taping a hose to his car's exhaust pipe. She said that he broke down crying and admitted that he was going to kill himself by carbon monoxide poisoning.

In addition, he has not been eating properly or tending to his self care. His weight has dropped from 185 pounds to 140 pounds over the past 6 months. His daughter has been very concerned because he refuses to check his glucose or take his insulin as recommended. She stated, "I think he was trying to kill himself by not taking care of his diabetes."

He is followed daily by your consult-liaison team, and his mental state improves each day. His MMSE score has improved to 28/30. On hospital day 5, the internal medicine team informs you that he has developed wet gangrene in his right lower extremity and will need to have a below-knee amputation as soon as possible. The team asks you to assess the patient's capacity to make medical decisions, because he is adamantly refusing to consent to this procedure.

You meet with the patient to discuss his medical situation. He is alert, lucid, and fully oriented. He states, "My doctor told me that I had an ulcer on my foot from poorly controlled diabetes that has become severely infected. I was told that I need to have my right leg amputated very soon or else I could die from the infection." He maintains that he is not interested in the surgical procedure

(continued)

that has been recommended. He added, "My daughter is begging me to have the surgery, but I'm already old and I don't want to have to use a prosthetic leg or a wheelchair. Ever since my wife passed away, all I have wished for is to die so I can join her in heaven."

Does this patient with severe major depressive disorder demonstrate the capacity to refuse a potentially life-saving procedure?

Yes, he demonstrates the capacity to refuse the recommended amputation. Legal standards for decision-making capacity to consent or refuse medical treatment involve the following: the ability to communicate a choice, to understand the relevant information, to appreciate the medical consequences of the situation, and to reason about treatment choices. In this case, the patient demonstrated the ability to discuss all of these topics. Although he was cognitively impaired on admission, his delirium eventually cleared.

The case is also complicated by the fact that the patient is currently suffering from major depression. Optimally, the consult liaison team may recommend treating the depression and readdressing the surgical procedure when his depression is in remission. However, this may take many weeks and failure to amputate the limb in a timely manner could result in death. Since the patient demonstrates decision-making capacity, the medical team must respect the patient's wishes and treat the condition without surgery.

Index

D

N

O

Q

R

S

T

U

V

W

X

Z

NOTES

NOTES

NOTES

NOTES

NOTES

NOTES

NOTES

NOTES

NOTES

NOTES